Ideology and social welfare

The Authors

Vic George is Professor of Social Policy and Administration and
Social Work at the University of Kent at Canterbury. Paul Wilding
is Professor of Social Administration at the University of
Manchester. Together they have written *Motherless Families* (1972),
Ideology and Social Welfare (1976) and *The Impact of Social Policy*
(1984), all published by Routledge & Kegan Paul. They were also
joint editors of the *Concepts in Social Policy* series (also published
by Routledge & Kegan Paul).

Radical Social Policy

GENERAL EDITOR:

Vic George

*Professor of Social Policy and
Administration and Social Work
University of Kent*

Ideology and social welfare

Completely revised, expanded and updated

Vic George
*Professor of Social Policy and
Administration and Social Work
University of Kent*

and

Paul Wilding
*Professor of Social Administration
University of Manchester*

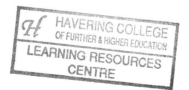

ROUTLEDGE

London and New York

First published 1985
by Routledge & Kegan Paul

Reprinted 1989
by Routledge
11 New Fetter Lane, London EC4P 4EE

Simultaneously published in the USA and Canada
by Routledge
a division of Routledge, Chapman and Hall, Inc.
29 West 35th Street, New York, NY 10001

Reprinted 1991

Printed in Great Britain by Guernsey Press

British Library Cataloguing in Publication Data
also available

Library of Congress Cataloging in Publication Data
George, Victor.
Ideology and social welfare.
(Radical social policy)
Bibliography: p.
Includes index.
I. Social policy 2. Welfare state. 3. Social
justice. I. Wilding, Paul. II. Title. III. Series.
HN16.G46 1985   361.6'1   84-27726

ISBN 0-415-05101-0

If we speak of democracy, we do not mean democracy which maintains the right to vote but forgets the right to work and the right to live. If we speak of freedom, we do not mean a rugged individualism which excludes social organisation and economic planning. If we speak of equality, we do not mean a political equality, nullified by social and economic privilege. If we speak of economic reconstruction, we think less of maximum production (though this too will be required) than of equitable distribution.

The Times, 1 July 1940

Contents

Acknowledgments

The first edition of *Ideology and Social Welfare* received both favourable and unfavourable comment from reviewers and other writers. We have benefited from that. Particularly helpful, however, has been the work of a number of writers on social policy whose work has appeared in recent years – Ian Gough, Ramesh Mishra, Robert Pinker, Graham Room, Peter Taylor-Gooby and Jennifer Dale.

We are grateful to Margaret Joyce at the University of Kent and to secretaries at the University of Manchester for typing several drafts of the manuscript.

Like all our other work this has been a truly collaborative effort and we are jointly responsible for any errors and shortcomings.

Introduction

When we wrote the earlier edition of this book in 1974 it was necessary to argue the case for studying the social values and the social and political ideas of those who write about social welfare. That is now no longer the case. The study of values and social theories has come to be seen as central to the understanding of social policies.

The structure of this revised book is the same as before. What we have done with each chapter is to review and revise it in the light of what has been written in recent years and in line with changes in our own ideas. Certainly, much has changed. The group we style the anti-collectivists has emerged from comparative obscurity to prominence in Britain and in other countries. New and important statements of anti-collectivist principles and practice have been published, though very few of them have been implemented by governments.

At the other end of the political spectrum there has been a great flowering of Marxist analysis of the nature and functions of public policy with particular emphasis on the notions of ideology and the state. Leaving aside the endless and often fruitless Byzantine debates among the various subdivisions of Marxism, this new literature has provided a more subtle structural framework for understanding the functions of the welfare state than the early Marxist analysis did.

In the middle ground there have been re-statements of the reluctant collectivist position – most powerfully from those within the Conservative Party who see the drift towards anti-collectivism as contrary to the traditional British Tory philosophy and practice. The new Social Democratic Party belongs to this school of thought even though its exponents have so far contributed little to the social policy debate.

Attacked from Right and Left and contaminated by actual experience of government, the Fabians have been on the defensive during the last ten years. It is only in the last couple of years that they have begun to rethink and restate their position in relation to economic and social policies seriously. Serious divisions of opinion still remain on several important aspects of public policy. Unity, however, exists on the parliamentary road to democratic socialism.

In the final chapter we attempt what we deliberately eschewed in 1974 – a comparison of the four perspectives reviewed in the book – as well as a clearer statement of our own theoretical position on the welfare state. In the earlier edition of this book we were rightly critical of the failures of the welfare state but failed both to defend its achievements and to say what should be done to make good the deficiencies. We attempt to put this right in the last few pages of this book by outlining the broad lines of a democratic socialist social policy strategy. It will, no doubt, be criticised as inadequate – and rightly so. Strategic thinking, however, has to begin somewhere and we hope we have made some contribution to it.

Vic George
University of Kent

Paul Wilding
University of Manchester

1

Society, the state, social problems and social policy

All advanced capitalist societies today are welfare states of a sort. They spend between one-third and one-half of their income on public services, half of which is taken up by what has come to be known as the social services. When this book was first written ten years ago, we noted that social policy was analysed as if it were an autonomous set of social institutions unconnected with the normal processes of the economic, social and political system in which it is set and which it serves. It is now, however, generally accepted that public and social services are part and parcel of the society in which they operate and an adequate understanding of their origin, aims and consequences necessitates an understanding of the nature of society.

Theories of society, of the state, of social problems and of social policy are inter-related. The view a social scientist holds of societal organisation and of the nature of the state will affect the explanation he or she gives of the incidence of social problems and of the government's response, if any, in the form of social policy measures. The link running through these four stages of conceptualisation is not always obvious nor does the relationship always correspond perfectly, but it nevertheless exists to a greater or lesser extent.

Any grouping of sociological and political theories inevitably oversimplifies what is essentially a very complex situation. It tends to emphasise unity rather than divergences of approach among theories belonging to the same group. Nevertheless, it has the important advantage of highlighting both the essential similarities and differences between the various groups and theories as well as their implications for social policy. It helps the development of a better understanding of the broad sweep of social policy at the cost perhaps of some oversimplification of the detailed aspects of social policy programmes.

Order, social conflict and class theories of society

The term 'order theories' is used here to include theories known in the sociological literature as order theories, consensus theories and functionalist theories. Obviously, there are differences of approach and emphasis among the sociologists of this broad school of thought but here only Parsons's views are used as they are so central to this school.[1] From the point of view of the present discussion, the central features of order theories of society are the stress on consensus, stability, integration and functional relations.[2] Every part of society is seen as having a specific function which contributes to the smooth running of society as a whole. In the early days of functionalism society was likened to a human body and the different subsystems of society to the different body organs. Though this analogy has long been abandoned by functionalist theorists, it illustrates the relationship between subsystems and society as a whole. When one part of society is out of line with the other parts there is pressure for its reintegration or for some realignment of other related parts. In this way, order and stability in society by and large prevail.

Social stability, however, according to these theorists, is based not simply on abstract functional necessity but on the real consensus of values that exists in society. Individuals share the same basic values and are thus agreed on how they should behave towards each other and on how society should operate. According to Parsons, the value system of society is 'the set of normative judgements held by members of society who define, with specific reference to their own society, what to them is a good society. . . . With all these qualifications, it is still true to say that values held in common constitute the primary reference point for the analysis of a social system as an empirical system.'[3] This general agreement on social values and behaviour patterns is perpetuated from one generation to the next through the twin processes of socialisation for the young and of social control for everyone.[4] As Lockwood rather tersely observes in his critique of Parsons, 'the two major threats to a given system are infants who have not been socialised and individuals who are motivated to deviance or non-conformity'.[5]

Clearly, explaining change in society does not come easily to order theories. Though allowance is made for change, it is seen as an aberration resulting from occasional dysfunctions in society or from technological change or outside pressures. The important point to make is that change is seen as an ephemeral phenomenon, perhaps a form of deviance, that is soon overcome, so that stability and order reign again in society. There are always adequate mechanisms built into the societal system to absorb the effects of any changes and to channel them into harmless processes. It is this claim for almost eternal stability that has provoked Gouldner's comment that 'Parsons has conceived of a social system that is immortal'.[6]

If little allowance is made for social change by functionalist theories, social conflict is considered almost abnormal and certainly harmful to society. The emphasis on consensus of values and behaviour patterns makes social conflict both very exceptional and detrimental to the interests of all in society. By implication, too, conflicts can be seen as deviant and disruptive. As Van den Berghe, a sympathetic critic of order theories has remarked: 'In so far as functionalists have had to take cognizance of problems of conflict and dissension, they have done so in terms of "deviance" or "variance", i.e. an unaccountable aberration from, or modification of, the "dominant pattern" which somehow tends to resolve itself through "institutionalization".'[7]

The emphasis and approval of consensus on one hand and the dismissal of conflict in society on the other, have rendered functionalism open to the criticisms of being a conservative view of society and of legitimising the *status quo*. An illustration of this criticism is the functionalist explanation of income and wealth inequalities in advanced industrial societies. Such inequalities, according to Davis and Moore, are not only inevitable because of the values prevailing in these societies but they are also beneficial to all in society. They act as a mechanism to ensure that the most vital positions in society are occupied by the most capable persons. If this were not to happen, economic growth and political stability would suffer to the detriment of all.[8] The second criticism relevant to this discussion of functionalism is that it does not square with the ongoing industrial conflicts, racial conflicts and gender conflicts that are characteristic of advanced industrial societies. It is for this reason that Inkeless has likened functionalism to 'a pair of rose coloured glasses which distort reality, screening out the harsh facts about conflict or purpose and interest in human affairs'.[9]

Social conflict and class conflict theories of society share a common perspective on the nature of advanced capitalist societies: individuals, groups and classes pursue their own interests and, in so doing, they are often in conflict with others. Conflict is seen as a fact of everyday life even though there are substantial differences of opinion about its origins, functions and methods of resolution. In Dubin's words, 'Conflict . . . is a reality with which social theorists must deal in constructing their general models of social behaviour.'[10]

The two main conflict schools of thought are Weberianism and Marxism – i.e. the social conflict and the class conflict schools. Weber saw industrial societies as being stratified along three dimensions: class, status and party. Class is defined in such a way that it refers to groups with common economic or material interests while status refers to groups with common life-styles and consumption patterns. Runciman expresses the difference between class and status well when he writes that 'class depends on where your money comes from and status on what it goes on'.[11] Class and status can overlap at times but they are distinct categories. By party Weber means not only political parties but also pressure and interest groups. Again, parties can overlap with classes and status groups but they are a distinct stratification category. In Weber's words, 'they need be neither purely class nor purely status parties; in fact, they are likely to be mixed types and sometimes they are neither'.[12]

In contrast to the structural-functionalist school which sees order as the inevitable outcome of the 'needs' of the social system, Weberianism adopts an action frame of reference with groups of people pursuing their interests in diverse ways and groupings. As Lambert, Paris and Blackaby put it: 'Within the action frame of reference, conflicts, disagreements and clashes of interests are continuous, constant and real, given the variety of interests, beliefs and ideas which people have and given the variety of interactions and relationships.'[13] It is clear from this account of conflict in society that economic interests are only one – albeit important – element in social conflict. Racial, religious, prestige, professional and other sources of conflict are also important. But if the sources of conflict are diverse and numerous, the likelihood of resolving such conflicts within the capitalist system is high because many of them are not dependent on or related to the capitalist ownership of the means of production or distribution. Though conflict is natural in industrial societies, political stability is maintained, claims the Weberian school, through a variety of processes, the main one being the 'belief by subordinates in the legitimacy of their subordination'.[14]

The Marxist theory of class conflict differs from the Weberian approach in a variety of ways, the main one being that it sees class conflict as far more important in society than other forms of conflict. This is because class conflict stems from the production system which, Marxists claim, is the foundation on which the social, political and ideological systems depend. Changes in the production system affect the relationships between the two main classes as well as the degree and form of class conflict. They also affect other forms of conflict in society in complex ways which we discuss in Chapter 5. Class conflict has an historic role to play because it can lead to the very abolition of the capitalist system itself. In the Weberian school the main vehicle of social change is the increasing rationality and bureaucratisation that is inherent in advanced capitalist societies. Clearly, the notion of class has very different meanings to these two schools of conflict theory.

The relative political stability prevailing in capitalist societies is neither natural nor beneficial to all. It is not natural because Marxists see the social system of capitalist societies as conflict-ridden and changing rather than as the stable, integrated structure observed by functionalists. Moreover, Marxists see such stability as being in the interests of the capitalist class. It is the result of various factors – coercion, economic dependence by working-class people on their employers, improvements in material standards and, above all, the legitimation of dominant values. These values serve the interests of the powerful groups in society but they are transformed into national values and they come to be accepted by working-class people. Thus, the general consensus which prevails in society does not, as order theorists claim, benefit all sections of society alike but is, in the view of the Marxists, a major mechanism of class domination and exploitation.

These three main interpretations of the structure of capitalist societies imply different perceptions of the nature and distribution of power and hence of the state. It is to these that we now turn.

Pluralist, élitist and class theories of the state

Order theories of society are associated with consensus or with pluralist views of power. Parsons sees power in consensus terms and suggests that it is vested in the government by the public for the fulfilment of collective ends. Power 'is the capacity to mobilize the resources of the society for the attainment of goals

5

for which a general "public" commitment has been made, or may be made.' [15]

Perhaps less idealistic than Parsons's view of power is the related pluralist conception. Pluralism holds that political power is shared between private individuals, pressure groups and the state. There is no one group in society which is so powerful that it dominates other groups let alone the government. Concentration of power in one group upsets the equilibrium of society with the result that opposing groups are formed to restore the balance – Galbraith's notion of countervailing power.[16] The individual is not lost in the negotiations or arguments between groups and government because his voice is heard through his membership of particular groups and at general elections. Moreover, the prevailing consensus on the 'democratic creed', claims Dahl, acts as a check on groups or individuals who may, from time to time, act in an 'un-American' fashion.[17] It follows from this view of power distribution in an integrated stable society that the state is either an impartial arbiter of minor conflicts among groups or simply the instrument through which agreed and non-controversial policies are introduced to the benefit of all in society. The state is seen as serving the public interest in all its activities. This is its primary concern, and it has certainly both the will and the power to curtail sectional interests if and when they arise.

If order theories are at ease with Dahl's one-face view of power, Weberian conflict theories are more in line with the two-dimensional view of power put forward by Bachrach and Baratz. Power, according to this view, consists not only of the ability to win arguments around the negotiating table – the one-face view of power – but also of the ability to exclude from discussion issues which are crucial to the maintenance of one's advantage. It is in this way, claim Bachrach and Baratz, that the business community has managed to maintain its privileged position in society.[18]

A conflict view of the state will therefore acknowledge that some groups in society always exercise more power than others. These groups are sometimes referred to as élites, as in the classic discussion by Wright Mills of the tripartite nature of the power élite in the United States. The three different élites – the top business executives, the top military men and the top civil servants – are related by education and family background and share a common interest in maintaining the *status quo*. Their influence on the government has therefore been immense.[19]

Though there are strong and weak versions of the power élite thesis, its general implication is that the state, willingly or unwillingly, has to take note of the interests of the élite groups in society. The policies it pursues and the policies which it excludes from discussion are affected by the two-dimensional power of these groups. As we shall see in Chapter 4, Fabian thinking on the state is compatible with this analysis. In the social policy literature, Hall *et al.* best exemplify this theoretical approach. They accept Bachrach's and Baratz's conception of power and emphasise the importance which élites have in setting 'the limits of policy-making' as regards both policies which are introduced and policies which are not included in government plans. They also raise for discussion the immense and obvious problems involved in researching into the 'non-decisions' of governments.[20]

The Marxist view of power goes a step beyond the conflict view and seeks to establish the structural sources of conflict: it locates them within the relations of production. The differential possession of power by the two main classes and their allies stems from their differential position in the production system. The class that owns the means of production inevitably possesses a great deal of power. The working class possesses power through its organisations and because its labour is indispensable to the production system. Normally the power of the upper class dominates, though under certain economic circumstances the working class can increase its power to match and even surpass that of the capitalist class. Clearly, this is a structural view of power which tries to locate its source and the mechanisms of its distribution in society. The crucial question, however, is whether all forms of power emanate directly or indirectly from the economic system. Weberians and others contest this and there are also disagreements among Marxists about the precise relationship between the economic system and the other subsystems of society.

Marxists have dwelt on the notion of the state far more than other groups. Their views of the state are divided between those who see the state as a mere servant of the capitalist class and those who feel that the state can, under certain circumstances, override the opposition of the capitalist class. The first view tends to use a very broad definition of the state – what Althusser calls the ideological and the repressive apparatus of the state. This includes the police, the media, the family, the Church, the civil service, the army and the government.[21] Even the most left-wing of governments, according to this view, will find it impossible to impose its will on the capitalist class on important issues through the normal parliamentary channels. The second view holds that left-wing governments with the support of a strong working class can introduce and implement radical policies even though they acknowledge that there will be fierce opposition from the capitalist class at the local, national and international level.[22] In general, most Marxists will be sympathetic to Birnbaum's conclusion that property owners and managers have the ability 'if not to impose their will upon the state at least to block or severely limit programs adverse to their interests'.[23] This line of approach accepts that some legislative inroads have been made into the privileged terrain of the upper classes but that these inroads have been few, restricted in scope and have often been substantially modified in practice. The ruling class, it is argued, may have lost several battles but it has so far always been able to win the war.

Personal, institutional and structural theories of social problems

A theory which emphasises stability, order, equilibrium and the functional relationship between the various parts of society and which stresses the pluralistic distribution of power and the notion of the impartial state will clearly tend to look for the causes of social problems in the personal characteristics of the individuals concerned and to search for individualistic solutions. Thus, order theories of society see social problems primarily in terms of deviance, disorganisation and hereditary inadequacies.

The essential difference between deviance and disorganisation, according to two of the main advocates of this view of social problems – Nisbet and Merton – is that 'the type of social problem involved in disorganisation arises not from people failing to live up to the requirements of their social statuses as is the case with deviant behaviour, but from the faulty organisation of these statuses into a reasonably coherent social system'.[24] The main sources of social disorganisation are 'breakdowns in channels of effective communication between people in a social system', 'defects in the processes of socialisation', and 'faulty arrangements of competing social demands upon people'.[25]

Deviant behaviour covers both non-conformist behaviour and aberrant behaviour – a distinction between on the one hand behaviour which is open, unselfish and esteemed by its practitioners and on the other, behaviour which is concealed, practised for personal gain and which is even felt to be stigmatising by the practitioners themselves. Only aberrant behaviour is seen as leading to social problems though it is acknowledged that there is no definitive and permanent dividing line between the concepts of aberration and non-conformism. Stealing, drug addiction, poverty and so on are forms of aberrant behaviour – they are social problems; unusual hair styles, unorthodox religious beliefs, and so on are non-conformist forms of behaviour and they do not constitute social problems. It is also acknowledged that disorganisation can lead to aberrant forms of deviance, as for example, in the case of children brought up in families whose socialisation practices are faulty due to group characteristics – gypsies, large impoverished families, and so on.

The disorganisation-deviant view of social problems dominated social science thinking until the 1960s when it came under severe attack and other views also gained acceptance. One of the early critics of the functionalist view of social problems, C. Wright Mills, pointed out that the whole approach was based on the assumption that white, middle-class styles of living were the norm, while others were problematic. The advocates of this view, whom he labelled as 'social pathologists', were also apologists of the existing social order despite their social scientific protestations.[26]

Ryan adds a new aspect to the criticism of functionalist theories by denouncing them as the old ideology of 'blaming the victim' dressed up in modern social scientific jargon. The strong appeal of this approach, he claimed, stemmed from its ability to appear humane, constructive and promising without, at the same time, posing any real threat to the *status quo*. Using a psychological perspective, Ryan argues that a liberal, progressive person faced with the dilemma of having to reconcile inequalities which he/she condemns in theory with his/her own privileged position in society, resorts to the 'blaming the victim' formula. The liberal progressive 'cannot side with an openly reactionary, repressive position that accepts continued opposition and exploitation as the price of a privileged position for his own class. This is incompatible with his own morality and his basic political principles.'[27] On the other hand, he rejects the solution of radical change on the pretext of its being too extreme while in fact it is because such a change threatens his own privileged position. The result is a compromise solution that is acceptable to the psyche and which leaves the *status quo* unchanged.

With such an elegant formulation, the humanitarian can have it both ways. He can, all at the same time, concentrate his charitable interests on the defects of the victim, condemn the vague social and environmental stresses that produced the defect (some time ago), and ignore the continuing effect of victimizing social forces (right now). It is a brilliant ideology for justifying a perverse form of social action designed to change, not society, as one might expect, but rather society's victim.[28]

⟨In brief, the disorganisation-deviant view sees social problems as having little or no connection with the unequal distribution of resources in society. As a result, it seeks solutions in the treatment of individuals, families, or, at most, neighbourhoods, rather than in any major changes to the prevailing unequal socio-economic conditions. Anti-collectivists would espouse such a line. They see the real causes of what are conventionally defined as social problems as lying within individuals and as therefore not amenable to amelioration or solution through government action. Such action will, in fact, cause or exacerbate other problems through the disruption it causes to the spontaneous order of society.⟩

The institutional approach, based on the social conflict model of society, turns the light away from the individual and towards society in general in the search for the causes of social problems. The roots of social problems, it is argued, lie not so much in personal inadequacies but in the economic and social conditions in which people find themselves. Poverty is largely the result of low wages or low social security benefits; ill-health is the result of unhealthy working and living conditions; unemployment is the outcome of a private profit-maximising economic system, and so on. Conflict writers argue that the behaviour of individuals can only be explained adequately within this broader framework. Human beings are seen as primarily social beings, shaped largely by their socio-economic environment.

Since they see society as conflict-ridden rather than as orderly and integrated, conflict theorists accept greater cultural diversity and tend to question the legitimacy of generally accepted forms of behaviour. Horton, in a concise discussion of order and conflict theories of social problems, expresses the difference of approach well. 'The conflict theorist', he writes, 'invariably questions the legitimacy of existing practices and values; the order theorist accepts them as the standard of health.'[29] Hence, forms of behaviour which, from a consensus point of view, are considered as social problems may, from a conflict perspective, be accepted simply as another form of behaviour with no implications for public policy. Indeed, some of these different forms of behaviour may even be seen in positive terms as spearheading change.

Conflict theorists see social problems as the product of conflicts of interests and values among the various groups in society. Indeed, they disapprove of the term 'social problem' because of its clinical connotations which help to defuse what are essentially political issues. Rule expresses this point well when he argues that:

> Race, pollution, poverty, the cities – all of these so-called 'social problems' amount to contests between various groups over the control of desirable resources, including wealth, privilege and, above all, the application of political power. These issues turn on clashes of interest, and thus represent political conflicts. And yet, in the language of the prevailing coalition between government and social science, they are treated instead as social problems, as forms of 'social sickness'. My thesis is that this unwarranted application of clinical language to politics is misleading and dangerous. For it suggests that political conflicts can somehow be resolved a-politically, through the dispassionate intervention of experts instead of through political action. And this suggestion paves the way, in turn, for the imposition of partisan measures in the guise of non-political 'solutions' to 'social problems'.[30]

Conflict theorists will therefore perceive fewer traditional social situations as 'social problems' and they would prefer to call these situations 'social conflicts' rather than social problems. But they would go further to claim that some situations which are considered normal should instead be considered as conflict situations and hence should be added to the list of 'social problems'. In this they receive support even from a functionalist source – Merton's thesis that the definition of a situation as a social problem is related to the power structure of society:

> Social definitions of social problems have this in common with other processes in society: those occupying strategic positions of authority and power of course carry more weight than others . . . in identifying for the rest what are to be taken as significant departures from social standards. There is not a merely numerical democracy of judgement in which every man's approval is assigned the same voting power in defining a condition as a social problem.[31]

Conflict theorists could therefore argue, for example, that the

11

payment of low wages or the manufacture of unhealthy consumer goods by private enterprise for profit purposes are social problems. The only reason that they are not so recognised by government is because of the power of certain élites in society. It is a good illustration of the two faces of power concept, that powerful groups have the ability to exclude from public discussion issues that are central to their privileged position.

In brief, a conflict perspective on social problems raises serious questions about the structure of society. The study of social problems from a conflict perspective is, as Sykes insists, 'nothing less than the study of what is considered the satisfactory and unsatisfactory organisation of society, not in terms of minor concerns arousing momentary public indignation but in terms of the major elements of the social structure'.[32] The implication of this approach is that whereas some social problems can be solved or substantially reduced under capitalism, others cannot.

Marxists find the term 'social problems' as unacceptable, if not more so, as conflict theorists. Its only purpose is to cloud and mystify structural issues of inequality, oppression or alienation and turn them into individualistic issues of deviance or inadequacy. Referring to the concept of deviance, Liazos suggests that

we should banish the concept of 'deviance' and speak of oppression, conflict, persecution, and suffering. By focussing on the dramatic forms, as we do now, we perpetuate most people's beliefs and impressions that such 'deviance' is the basic cause of many of our troubles, that these people (criminals, drug addicts, political dissenters, and others) are the real 'troublemakers', and necessarily, we neglect conditions of inequality, powerlessness, institutional violence, and so on, which lie at the bases of our tortured society.[33]

It follows from their analysis of society that Marxists will see so-called social problems as the result not of industrialisation, urbanisation or conflicts between groups but as the result of the capitalist form of production and its accompanying forms of social relationships. For some social problems this explanation is direct and obvious; for others it is more complex and less obvious. Poverty is an example of the first category and crime of the second.

Poverty is the inescapable outcome of the private ownership of the means of production. Capitalists invest their capital to make profit and workers sell their labour for their livelihood. In this structurally determined conflict situation the level of wages not only affects the level of profitability but also takes no account of the individual worker's family needs. It is therefore inevitable that many working-class people will have incomes insufficient to meet their basic family needs. It is the natural outcome of this form of production relationship.

Crime is different from poverty because it is a form of behaviour rather than a type of condition. Nevertheless, crime too will be explained in terms of the capitalist system of production because all forms of behaviour are influenced and even determined by the economic structure. As Taylor *et al.* observe, Marx and Engels saw crime as an adjustment to the capitalist system rather than as a form of rebellion or insurrection. Moreover, they saw it neither as 'inevitable' nor as 'normal' forms of behaviour in any society.[34] They insisted that it was a feature of capitalism though they did not speculate that it would either disappear or substantially decline under socialism.

As we shall see later in this chapter, Marxists naturally maintain that since 'social problems' are in the last resort caused by the capitalist system, social policies in a capitalist society cannot hope to achieve very much.

Integration, truce and class theories of social policy

As we saw earlier in this chapter, a functionalist view of society implies that all the subsystems of society perform one or more functions which are necessary for society's orderly functioning. The social services are one of these societal subsystems and, though they perform economic and political functions, their main task is to promote social integration and the general acceptance of the basic values of society. They perform these functions in a general way and also in specific ways when they deal with particular deviant groups. They act at both a preventative and a treatment level. As with social problems, functionalists tend to see social policy in non-political, non-ideological and non-partisan terms. In reality, however, it is a view of social policy which has obvious conservative implications.

Historically, claim the functionalists, the social services developed as a result of the increased differentiation and specialisation in society brought about by industrialisation. Industrialisation resulted in migration from rural to urban areas; it meant the total dependence of people on paid employment for their livelihood; it had the effect of modifying the extended family and its traditional roles; it necessitated new forms of industrial training; it created new health problems through unplanned massive urbanisation and factory employment, and so on. These changes inevitably meant that the traditional institutions for providing social welfare – the family, the guilds, the Church, the voluntary agencies – could not cope. Statutory social services thus became necessary and governments responded by providing such services. There was a functional need for social services and it was natural and inevitable that governments would respond in order to restore integration and stability in society to the benefit of everyone.

Since industrialisation has affected all countries, it has meant that the same changes and the same responses to these changes have taken place in all industrial countries. The welfare state is thus a stage of societal development through which all industrial countries go.[35] But more than that – the welfare state has created a consensual society. It is, at the same time the product of societal consensus about ends and means and contributes to such a consensus. It has contributed to 'the end of ideology', to use Bell's words. In the Western world, he claimed in the early 1960s, 'there is today a rough consensus among intellectuals on political issues: the acceptance of a welfare state; the desirability of decentralised power; a system of a mixed economy and of political pluralism'.[36] The reason for this is that the main issues and problems have been resolved and what remains is an assortment of trifling questions which can be settled through judicious piecemeal social engineering. Parsons expressed this view equally strongly: 'Through industrial development, under democratic auspices', he claimed, 'the most important legitimately to-be-expected aspirations of the "working class" have in fact been realised.'[37]

No one will quarrel with the claim that industrialisation brought about numerous changes in society and created new problems. Conflict, Marxist and other theories obviously accept this. It is the functionalist explanation of social policy development that is unacceptable to the other theories. The main weaknesses of functionalist explanations are to be found in their three claims that social policy is functionally necessary and hence 'inevitable' in its origins; that it is 'neutral' and hence 'generally beneficial' in its consequences; and that it is universal and hence similar in pattern in all industrial countries. Goldthorpe wrote of the first and second weaknesses that

A functionalist explanation of the development of social policy requires to be refined and supplemented through analysis which takes an 'action' frame of reference; that is analysis in terms of the ends of individuals and groups rather than in terms of the 'needs' of society considered as a whole.[38]

A functionalist explanation, however, which takes into account such an action frame of reference ceases to be functionalist.

Similarly, the claim that social policy measures are broadly similar in all industrial societies is disputed. The fact that industrial societies may accept responsibility for the provision of a service or spend similar proportions of their resources on the same service does not necessarily mean that they provide a similar social service from the point of view of the recipients. Even when some functionalist writers concede that there are variations in the social services of different industrial countries, their theoretical approach cannot adequately explain these variations. Finally, the recent party political disputes on the role of social services and the election of governments with a residual approach to social policy have seriously strained the credibility of functionalism as an explanatory model of the development and role of social policy.[39] The only lasting merit of the functionalist approach to social policy is that it seeks to explain its development as part of ongoing economic and social change in society.

Anti-collectivists do not see the development of social policy as functional to the development of capitalism or to social stability. In fact they see an extended role for the state in welfare as threatening to the economic and social well-being of a free market economy. The welfare state, in their view, has developed through the misguided efforts of individuals and groups to remedy particular problems. Short-term solutions have been devised, applied and accepted without much thought to the long-term consequences. Individuals are frequently well-meaning in their intentions, groups are self-interested.

The conflict approach to social policy flows naturally from the view that society is made up of classes and groups with conflicting interests; that these groups possess differential power and their influence on the state varies accordingly; and that though the actions of the state are grossly influenced, they are not totally controlled by the power of the strongest élites in society.

Conflict theorists, therefore, will see social policy measures as fundamentally the result of conflicts between various groups in society. Governments may be pressurised into introducing social policy legislation; or governments may be elected in order to introduce such legislation; but in both cases the type of legislation introduced will bear the marks of such conflicts. Hall *et al.* adopt this line of explanation:

> Social policy is partly a history of conflict between interests; interests which have often been concentrated in different social classes. But it is also and even more clearly a history of conflicts being resolved, of accommodation, compromise and of agreements which cut across class boundaries.[40]

Rex adopts a similar approach but from a wider conceptual perspective. Conflicts between classes, groups or political parties in society can be resolved, he argues, in one of three ways: in the interests of the ruling class; in the interests of the oppressed or exploited group; or in compromises which modify the position of the ruling group through some concessions to the oppressed group. These compromises, which he calls truce situations, are characteristic of the outcomes of conflicts in welfare states. Truce situations are, by their very nature, unstable situations and they are always open to renegotiation but they 'could only become the basis of a new social order in exceptionally favourable conditions'.[41] In other words, welfare state measures are neither mere props to the capitalist system nor socialist measures but, rather, they potentially confer some benefit on all groups in society though not necessarily equal benefit. It is to be expected, however, that the most powerful groups will manage to make use of the best schools, or the best health service facilities. Instead of the conflict taking place in the market place, it now 'takes place immediately at the political level' but with similar results.[42] Even within a service provided only for working-class people, such as public housing, the more powerful groups manage to get the best of what is available with the result that weak groups such as immigrants or one-parent families receive the worst. Thus 'housing classes', 'education classes', etc., emerge, reflecting new political groupings in a society where such goods are provided by the state rather than the private market. Though they sometimes overlap with groupings produced by the private market, they nevertheless create a far more complex pattern of power distribution than that envisaged by the simple Marxist social class model.

Because of their view of the state, most conflict theorists maintain that left-wing governments can introduce legislation which can deal with such problems as poverty, inadequate housing and the like. Such measures will be resisted by the upper classes but the state is not simply a servant of the capitalist class,

16

as the Marxists claim.

Chapter 5 discusses in some detail the Marxist view of the welfare state and, therefore, only the bare outline is presented here. The growth of social services is seen as being the result, primarily, of two processes in society: conflict between the two main classes and the needs of the capitalist system. The class conflict model adopts an action frame of reference similar to the truce situation model but it makes classes rather than groups the central agents of change. Governments are directly or indirectly pressurised by the working class to introduce social policy legislation though the character of the legislation will take into account the inevitable opposition from the capitalist class. In this way, though social reforms represent the triumphs of working-class struggles, they do not necessarily benefit the working class more than the capitalist class.

Social reforms may also be introduced to 'meet the needs of capitalism' – to make the capitalist system more efficient or more acceptable to the working class and hence more stable. It follows from such an analysis that the main, ultimate beneficiary of social reforms is the capitalist class. Several attempts have been made by Marxists to combine and reconcile the 'class conflict' and the 'needs of capitalism' approach with varying degrees of success.[43]

In the end, however, in capitalist welfare states a situation is reached where public expenditure outruns the government's ability to raise the necessary revenues. This is a structural tendency, which O'Connor calls the fiscal crisis of the state. It has little to do with administrative inefficiency or other bureaucratic factors.[44] When such a situation is created, the state will attempt to reduce public expenditure but, by so doing, it runs the risk of undermining either capital profitability or political stability or both. The only real solution is the abolition of the capitalist system and the creation of a socialist society where both profits and social expenses are managed by the government to the benefit of all.

It follows from this brief description of the Marxist model that, according to this perspective, social policy cannot solve the fundamental 'social problems' of capitalist society. Thus Miliband, whilst accepting that social reforms have benefited the working class and the poor, maintains that poverty cannot be abolished in a capitalist system: '. . . the truth – the bitter truth – is that the abolition of poverty', he insists, 'will have to wait until the abolition of the system which breeds it comes on the agenda; and this is a question which far transcends the issue of poverty itself.'[45] Similarly, crime cannot be abolished under capitalism, claims Quinney, because working-class crimes 'are actually a means of *survival*, an attempt to exist in a society where survival is not assured by other, collective means. Crime is inevitable under capitalist conditions.'[46]

This chapter has reviewed briefly the positions of the three main groups of theorists on the nature of society, of social problems, of the state, and of social policy in advanced industrial societies. These issues will be elaborated and illustrated further in the chapters that follow.

2

The anti-collectivists

Anti-collectivism was the dominant ideology in nineteenth-century Britain, but in the last years of the century it was increasingly challenged. In the twentieth century, it lapsed into academic and political obscurity – particularly in the years between 1940 and 1970. The recession which overtook many of the advanced industrial countries from the early 1970s, however, encouraged a resurgence of anti-collectivist thought. Its advocates – Hayek, Friedman, the Institute of Economic Affairs, for example – gained a new eminence and influence. Ten years ago it was possible to regard anti-collectivism as an interesting but rather quaint anachronism. That is no longer possible. It is vigorously alive and academically and politically influential.

Social values

Freedom, individualism and inequality are the fundamental social values of the anti-collectivists. They make up the core of the anti-collectivist value system.

Freedom or liberty – and anti-collectivists generally use the terms interchangeably – is the basic value. 'As liberals,' says Friedman, 'we take freedom of the individual, or perhaps the family, as our ultimate goal in judging social arrangements.'[1] Hayek gives it an equal priority. 'Liberty', he wrote in 1961, 'is not just one value among others, a maxim of morality on a par with all maxims, but the source of, a necessary condition for, all other individual values.'[2] As such, freedom must be recognised as an absolute principle. It will prevail, Hayek argues, 'only if it is accepted as a general principle whose application to particular instances requires no justification'.[3] This will mean 'a constant rejection of measures which appear to be required to secure particular results, on no stronger ground than that they conflict with a general rule'[4] – the principle of liberty.

What is this freedom? It is an essentially negative state – the absence of coercion. Freedom is maximised when coercion is reduced as much as possible in society. What is this coercion? Hayek defines it as 'such control of the environment or circumstances of a person by another that . . . he is forced to act not according to a coherent plan of his own but to serve the ends of another'. The essential evil of such coercion is that it individual as a thinking and valuing person and bare tool in the achievement of the ends of

One point this definition of coercion is of critical importance to an understanding of the anti-collectivist view of the world. It is specific human agencies acting with intent can act in a which appropriately defined as coercive. Hayek argues for example, that even if compelled by the threat of starvation to take an unpleasant job at a very low wage a man or woman is not coerced because no one intended that he or she should be compelled to serve someone else's ends.[6]

Why is freedom so centrally important to anti-collectivists? Firstly, they see freedom quite simply as a natural right, something to which all individuals have a *prima facie* claim by virtue of their common humanity. Secondly, their emphasis on freedom reflects the anti-collectivists' critical assessment of human limitations of knowledge and character. If there were men who were omniscient, Hayek argues, there would be little case for liberty. It is because men are ignorant and because 'we rarely know which of us knows best that we trust the independent and competitive efforts of many to induce the emergence of what we shall want when we see it'.[7] Freedom makes it possible to use much more knowledge than the mind of the wisest ruler or best informed government could make available. Making freedom the primary value also places restraints on the natural inclination of men to oppress other men – albeit in their best interests.

The third reason for the anti-collectivist stress on freedom is its inter-relationship with a market economy. The market both requires freedom and is a powerful element in its preservation.

As Friedman puts it 'the central feature of the market organisation of economic activity is that it prevents one person from interfering with another in respect of most of his activities'.[8] But the market cannot operate in this beneficent way unless individuals are free and uncoerced to start with.

Finally, freedom is seen as a necessary and sufficient means to a wide variety of desirable ends. For Hayek, 'the only moral principle which has ever made the growth of an advanced civilisation possible was the principle of individual freedom'.[9] Friedman is even more rapturous:

> A society that puts freedom first will, as a happy byproduct, end up with both greater freedom and greater equality. . . . A free society releases the energies and abilities of people to pursue their own objectives. It prevents some people from arbitrarily suppressing others. . . . It preserves the opportunity for today's disadvantaged to become tomorrow's privileged and, in the process, enables almost everyone, from top to bottom, to enjoy a fuller and richer life.[10]

The anti-collectivists are aware that taking freedom as their primary value does create problems. The judgment in favour of freedom is one of balance. Freedom gives people the opportunity to do things which will be regarded as undesirable. That has to be accepted. So too does the fact that 'the preservation of individual freedom is incompatible with a full satisfaction of our ideas of distributive justice'.[11] Freedom means that some people will seem to be treated less than fairly. That is the cost to be set against the other manifold gains.

When set against some of its immediate costs freedom will not always be popular because the longer-term gains will, by definition, be less obvious than some of the short-term costs. As Brogan put it, 'political liberty is not the only, perhaps not the main demand made by the average man on society'.[12] Men have to be persuaded that on balance, and over time, the gains of pursuing freedom outweigh the costs.

The second fundamental value for the anti-collectivists is individualism. It is complementary to freedom and neither can exist without the other. A free society, they argue, will promote individualism, and a strong sense of individualism makes unnecessary or impossible large-scale state intervention or coercion.

Individualism is two things. Firstly, it is a theory of society, an attempt, as Hayek puts it, 'to understand the forces which determine the social life of men'.[13] The theory holds that social phenomena can only be understood through an understanding of the actions of individuals. It rejects the notion that societies can be understood 'as entities *sui generis* which exist independently of the individuals which compose them'.[14] It sees the individual as the vital factor in economic and social development rather than forces, trends or evolutionary processes.

Secondly, individualism is a set of political maxims about how society should be organised, derived from and contributing to a particular view of the state. The primary maxim is that much which is currently undertaken by the state would be better undertaken by individuals.

Individualism sees men as irrational, self-centred and fallible. Where individual action rather than government policy is the norm the errors of individuals are corrected by social processes. One man's ignorance and fallibility does not become dominant. Through interaction, individuals' actions are modified, corrected and supplemented and achievements are produced beyond the capacities of any individual. As Hayek puts it the 'spontaneous collaboration of free men often creates things which are greater than their individual minds can ever comprehend'.[15] Competition, even by imperfect and irrational men, is a surer road to progress than is action by the state.

Individualism also leads to a particular theory of economic development and to particular prescriptions for economic policy. Mrs Thatcher has argued that economic development in the Western world has been more rapid because the moral philosophy is superior. 'It is superior', she insists, 'because it starts with the individual, with his uniqueness, his responsibility and his capacity to choose.'[16] The belief that if the individual is freed from state interference and given proper incentives economic development will be facilitated is a basic article of faith for anti-collectivists.

Individualism is also seen as a prerequisite of a responsible society. Hayek makes this point in his indictment of the effects of 'the predominance of the idea of the "social" '. He believes that the effect has been 'the destruction of the feeling of personal responsibility to which it has led'.[17] More directly, he argues that 'responsibility to be effective must be individual responsibility'.[18] Mrs Thatcher urges individualism as the basis of what she styles 'The Healthy Society' – 'a society in which the vast majority of men and women are encouraged and helped to accept responsibility for themselves and their families, and to live their lives with a maximum of independence and self reliance'.[19] The citizens of such a healthy society 'are people who care for others and look first to themselves to care for themselves'.[20]

The final political maxim to be derived from individualism is that many conditions described by commentators with other values as social problems, because socially caused, are more properly seen as problems with individual causes. The political implication of this view is that such problems and conditions can only be remedied by individual action and individual change and not by government policy. As the key to Mrs Thatcher's success in promoting the new economic liberalism Gamble describes 'the posing of central questions of government policy as problems of individual responsibility and individual choice'.[21]

The third central value held by anti-collectivists is inequality. It is closely connected with their repudiation of the notion of social justice but we will deal with inequality first. The basis of the anti-collectivist belief in inequality is the view that the pursuit of egalitarian policies is incompatible with freedom. In Friedman's words 'one cannot be both an egalitarian . . . and a liberal'.[22] The pursuit of equality would make inevitable a range of policies quite unacceptable to anyone with a primary commitment to freedom. Hayek writes of equality of the general rules of law and conduct – civil and political rights – as 'the only kind of equality conducive to liberty and the only equality which we can secure without destroying liberty'.[23] The essence of his objection to egalitarian policies is that a demand for equality is 'the professed motive of most of those who desire to impose upon society a preconceived pattern of distribution' and he objects to all such attempts 'whether it be an order of equality or of inequality'.[24] The desirability of a particular objective can never justify the use of coercion.

The anti-collectivists also put forward pragmatic arguments in favour of inequality. They stress the economic benefits which accrue from the incentives to innovation and effort which inequality generates. Sir Keith Joseph wrote in 1976 that redistribution in Britain had reached the point at which it was 'actually reducing national wealth by discouraging wealth creators'.[25] Hayek speaks of rapid economic advance as 'in a large measure' the result of inequality and 'impossible without it'.[26] Sir Keith neatly sums up the argument about freedom leading inescapably to inequality, and inequality bringing economic gains in his conclusion that 'the pursuit of income equality will turn this country into a totalitarian slum'. It will endanger 'freedom, prosperity and the prospect for eliminating poverty'.[27] In Milton Friedman's judgment, British domestic policy since 1945 'has been dominated by the search for greater equality of outcome'. 'Who can doubt the effect', he asks in complete confidence about the response of the intelligent reader, 'that the drive for equality has had on efficiency and productivity? Surely that is one of the main reasons why economic growth in Britain has fallen so far behind its continental neighbours, the United States, Japan and other nations over the past few decades.'[28] Inequality then is economically beneficial to society.

Another powerful argument favoured by anti-collectivists against policies for greater equality is their damaging social effects. Hayek describes egalitarianism as 'the most destructive of the constructivist morals'.[29] This is because he sees egalitarianism as leading to coercive policies and the breakdown of restraint in society. The result is the weakening of curbs on the rapacious instincts of all groups who want more for themselves.[30] Differences are no longer accepted. As they are debated so grievances are fuelled and social cohesion is threatened. Joseph and Sumption, for example, argue that cohesion is not necessarily destroyed by inequality but is inevitably destroyed by the abrasive measures required to make men equal.[31]

Milton Friedman paints an even more alarming picture of the social costs of egalitarian policies. Most people, he suggests, do not believe in 'the drive for equality' which has been such a feature of British domestic policy.[32] Because they do not believe in egalitarian policies, they evade or break the relevant laws. Lack of respect for law is infectious. It spreads even to those laws that 'everyone regards as moral and proper – laws against violence, theft and vandalism'. 'Hard as it may be to believe' he continues, and indeed belief is not entirely easy, 'the growth of crude criminality in Britain in recent decades may well be one consequence of the drive for equality.'[33]

What the anti-collectivists oppose is attempts to further or secure equality of outcome. Three other kinds of equality they find quite acceptable – equality of general rules, that is that laws apply to all citizens equally – equality of civil and political rights – and equality of opportunity. 'Equality of general rules of law and conduct', Hayek writes, 'is the only kind of equality conducive to liberty and the only equality we can secure without destroying liberty.'[34] Equality of opportunity is seen by Friedman as 'an essential component of liberty'[35] and by Joseph and Sumption as 'the corollary of the liberty of the individual'.[36] It is acceptable because it does not presuppose any particular social arrangements as desirable.

It is impossible to conclude a discussion of the fundamental values of anti-collectivism without exploring Hayek's view on social justice which is a continuing theme in his work. For Hayek the term social justice is 'entirely empty and meaningless'[37] for a number of reasons. First and foremost, he insists that a state of affairs can only be described as just or unjust if it was deliberately willed and contrived by an individual. As long as society remains a spontaneous order the particular results of the social process cannot reasonably be described as just or unjust. Hayek readily admits that if the pattern of allocation of goods and services which results from the market system was the result of a deliberate, planned pattern of allocation it would have to be regarded as very unjust. Since, however, what people receive is not the outcome of a planned process the results cannot be described as just or unjust.[38]

It is an illusion too, Hayek argues, to think that governments can pursue policies predicated on an ideal of social justice. Such an ideal 'presupposes an agreement on the relative importance of the different concrete ends which cannot exist in a great society whose members do not know each other or the same particular facts'.[39]

Another major objection to the notion of social justice is the way in which it is in conflict with freedom. A policy of social justice would necessitate strong direction by a central authority. This leads Hayek to assess the current belief in social justice as 'probably the gravest threat to most other values of a free civilisation'[40] and as 'the Trojan Horse through which totalitarianism has entered'.[41]

The desire for social justice is not difficult to understand. It is part of 'the atavistic craving for visible common purposes' which characterised the small group society of the past but is incompatible with the spontaneous order of the Great Society where all that is possible is agreement about means not ends.[42] But the desire shows a failure to grasp the nature of the spontaneous order and the impossibility of tinkering with any of its parts – in this case essentially the distribution of income and wealth – without disrupting its delicate patterns of self-regulation.

Friedman provides a much simplified version of Hayek's argument though he writes of 'fairness' rather than 'social justice'. He makes the essential points – the problem of who is to decide what constitutes fairness, the 'fundamental conflict' between the ideal of fair shares and the ideal of personal liberty, the way in which a government policy for fair shares can increase rather than moderate economic and social discontent, the benefits which accrue 'from the very unfairness we deplore'.[43]

If the term 'social justice' is empty of meaning then there can be no policy of redistribution by government. Equality has already been condemned and rejected by the anti-collectivists. 'Social Justice' might have provided a softer, more flexible guideline. Its rejection leaves no logical scope for a modification of the patterns of distribution delivered by the spontaneous order.

Society and the state

We consider the attitudes of our chosen thinkers to society and the state under five headings – their view of societal organisation in general, their views of the economic, social and political system and their view of the state.

The anti-collectivists do not have a straightforward consensus or conflict model of society because they are concerned primarily with individuals and individual action rather than with structures and structural forces. They are clear that societal agreement about ends is impossible and that attempts to secure it will simply be divisive. On the other hand, they are confident that agreement can be secured about how the society should run – the general rules. The fact that they have no hope of agreement about ends shows that their model is fundamentally a conflict one, but they stress conflict between individuals, which they describe as competition and see as having desirable effects for individuals and for society. Where anti-collectivists emphasise the strength of conflicts of interest in society they see such conflict as based on group rather than class interests.

The anti-collectivists – Hayek in particular – stress the central function of law in the maintenance of societal organisation in a free society. Hayek makes the distinction between a free, law-governed society – a nomocratic society as he calls it – and an unfree, telocratic or purpose-governed social order striving after some model of desirable social arrangements.[44]

The anti-collectivists' view of the economic system is basic to their whole philosophy. Liberalism, writes Hayek, derives, 'from the discovery of a self generating or spontaneous order in social affairs . . . an order which made it possible to utilise the knowledge and skill of all members of society to a much greater extent than would be possible in any order created by central direction'.[45]

What is the basis of this economic order? Essentially it is economic forces working in free competition and competition is a better way of guiding individual efforts than any other, and it is 'the only method by which our activities can be adjusted to each other without coercive or arbitrary intervention of authority'.[46] Competition makes possible an economic order much more complex than anything that could be created through central planning or direction.

> It was men's submission to the impersonal forces of the market that in the past has made possible the growth of a civilisation without which this could not have developed; it is by thus submitting that we are every day helping to build something that is greater than anyone of us can fully comprehend.[47]

The anti-collectivists develop an elaborate case for the free market economy. They are convinced of the general principle that in Bosanquet's words, 'the pursuit of the selfish aims of the individual will usually lead him to serve the general interest'.[48] They see the market system as a vital bulwark of political freedom because it means no group in society controls both economic and political power. As Friedman puts it, 'by removing the organisation of economic activity from the control of political authority, the market eliminates this source of coercive power. It enables economic strength to be a check to political power, rather than a reinforcement'.[49] 'Economic freedom is an essential requisite for political freedom.'[50]

The free market is also regarded as the most efficient way to organise an economy. Sir Keith Joseph's tributes are perhaps the most eloquent but differ only in degree from those of Hayek or Friedman.

> The blind, unplanned, uncoordinated wisdom of the market . . . is overwhelmingly superior to the well researched, rational, systematic, well meaning, cooperative, science-based, forward looking, statistically respectable plans of governments . . . the market system is the greatest generator of national wealth known to mankind: coordinating and fulfilling the diverse needs of countless individuals in a way which no human mind or minds could ever comprehend, without coercion, without direction, without bureaucratic interference.[51]

The market attains this level of efficiency because it is the best way of making use of what Bosanquet describes as 'dispersed knowledge' – the knowledge of all consumers and producers.[52]

27

Through the market mechanism efforts are coordinated without coercion. Producers and consumers are linked to their mutual benefit through competition and the price mechanism. Competition is not only 'in most circumstances the most efficient method known [of coordinating individual efforts], but even more because it is the only method by which our activities can be adjusted to each other without coercive or arbitrary intervention of authority'.[53]

The market mechanism is also the most efficient way of organising economic activity because it is, in Enoch Powell's words, the 'unique key' with which 'to unlock imprisoned energies',[54] and encourages experiment in a way which a planned economy cannot rival. It rewards success and punishes failure. It is the best method yet devised for registering preferences. As Friedman puts it 'it gives people what they want instead of what a particular group thinks they ought to want'.[55]

The proof of the pudding, of course, is in the eating. The anti-collectivists are convinced that the market system is the great engine of economic growth making possible a more sophisticated, complex, efficient and responsive economy. 'Wherever the free market has been permitted to operate', Friedman argues, ' . . . the ordinary man has been able to attain levels of living never dreamed of before.'[56] Hayek argues on similar lines that the market system serves the ends of every citizen 'by increasing the prospects or chances of everyone of a greater command over the various goods (i.e. commodities and services) than we are able to secure in any other way'.[57]

Friedman indignantly repudiates the 'myth' that free market capitalism is 'a system under which the rich exploit the poor'.[58] On the contrary 'the greater achievements of Western capitalism have redounded primarily to the benefits of the ordinary person'.[59] Hayek argues more specifically about how the market has helped the poorest. 'It has been this market mechanism', he insists, 'which has created the increase of aggregate income which also has made it possible to provide outside the market for the support of those unable to earn enough.'[60]

The market system is not simply a way of running a country's economic affairs. It is also a profound influence on the broader social system. One of Hayek's great insights was to set the study of market relationships in the broader context of social, political and legal relationships. He stresses the way the market bonds people socially by linking them in direct economic relationships and makes possible the peaceful reconciliation of divergent purposes. In Hayek's view, 'that interdependence of all men,

28

which is now in everybody's mouth and which tends to make all mankind One World, not only is the effect of the market order but could not have been brought about by any other means'.[61]

Seldon has recently added a new defence of the market, that 'market failure is essentially corrigible. Government failure is incorrigible.'[62] His argument is that the essential market principles are sound although to function effectively some differences in purchasing power may need to be corrected. On the other hand, if the market system is replaced by political decisions about the distribution of goods and services it is much more difficult to correct the inequalities of political power which will determine who gets what in that system of allocation.

Despite their confidence in the market system the anti-collectivists see it as an essentially delicate and fragile system. One of Hayek's chief anxieties is over the temptation which afflicts all governments to intervene at particular points to improve its functioning or to achieve a supposedly more desirable pattern of distribution. He accepts the strength of the temptation but condemns it for the lack of understanding of the spontaneous order which it reveals. 'It is not in our power', he writes, 'to build a desirable society by simply putting together the particular elements that by themselves appear desirable.'[63] The preservation of a spontaneous, market order is so difficult precisely because it requires a constant rejection of measures which appear to be required to secure particular, desirable results.[64]

At the heart of anti-collectivist concerns about the health of the market is concern about levels of public expenditure. According to simple anti-collectivist principles 'We are now on a road to serfdom with a speedometer marked by the percentages of GNP devoted to state welfare services'.[65] That speedometer also marks out the stages on the road to economic ruin. The argument is eminently simple. High levels of public expenditure demand high rates of taxation, which remove the incentive for harder work or new initiatives and drain industry of the money needed for working capital and new investment. To meet the inevitable shortfall in its needs, because no government likes raising taxes, governments committed to high levels of public spending will be driven to heavy borrowing. Interest rates will then rise and companies will find it even more difficult to raise capital. Inflation follows as individuals seek to make good the ravages of the taxman through pay increases.

The result, in Mrs Thatcher's words, is 'a sense of despair and hopelessness among our wealth creators'.[66] In the face of these body blows the economy fails to continue to deliver the golden eggs of growth. To quote Mrs Thatcher again, 'Taxation and inflation have damaged the stability and framework of order necessary to accommodate genuine economic expansion and social change'.[67] In Hayek's view, the spectacular legal privileges granted to the trade unions in the Trade Disputes Act 1906 have so upset a free market in labour as to become 'the chief cause of the progressive decline of the British Economy'.[68]

Because the anti-collectivists see the free market system as operating for the benefit of all, they see society as fundamentally healthy and stable so long as the delicacy of the spontaneous order is accepted. Economic freedom, says Friedman, 'preserves the opportunity for today's disadvantaged to become tomorrow's privileged and, in the process, enables almost everyone, from top to bottom, to enjoy a fuller and richer life'.[69] Society will be stable because the market system offers freedom and 'a constantly rising set of minimum standards – including rising minimum standards of income'.[70] Anti-collectivists see the biggest danger to social stability as lying in conflict between interest groups. Growth of the sphere of government action has led to the proliferation of organised groups seeking their own interests which can only be furthered at the expense of the rest of society. Of all such groups the government bureaucracy is in some ways the most powerful and dangerous.[71]

What of anti-collectivist views of the political system? In *The Constitution of Liberty* Hayek sets out what he regards as the three chief arguments for democracy 'each of which may be regarded as conclusive'. They are that democracy is the only way of resolving differences peacefully, that it is an important safeguard of individual liberty, and that it is the best way of educating people about public affairs.[72]

But Hayek had less confidence in democracy than he had in the processes of the spontaneous order. 'We have no ground', he wrote a few pages later, 'for crediting majority decision with that higher, super-individual wisdom which, in a certain sense, the products of spontaneous social growth may possess.'[73] It is the fact that majority decisions tell us what people want at a given moment rather than what would be in their real interests to want if they were better informed which troubles Hayek.[74] The basic problem is the potential impact of majority decisions on the present and future functioning of the spontaneous order.

The problematic relationship between democracy and economic and social stability has become a major theme in anti-collectivist writing. In essence the problem is that democracy tends to generate pressures and demands which are incompatible

30

with a market order. Competition between parties leads to competitive bidding for votes. The result of this process is to impart 'a systematic upward bias to expectations'.[75] Electors are offered much – all of it highly desirable in an ideal world. There is little discussion of how it is to be paid for or of the inevitability of choice. An excessive burden is thus placed on government expenditure and on the 'sharing out' function of government.[76] Hayek's analysis is very similar. Democracy, he believes, has spawned the entirely false notion that the powers of majority government are unlimited. This leads majorities into all kinds of new fields of activity in an effort to buy and retain the support of potential voters. In the search for short-term party gains the spontaneous order is threatened.

Democracy has led to the abandonment of the tacit belief that the sphere of government should be limited. The spontaneous order depends for its survival, however, on governments refusing to interfere with particular aspects of its functioning, a pattern of self-denial by governments to which democracies with a belief in unlimited government are strangers. The spontaneous order does not depend on design; it depends on the free decisions of innumerable individuals. Its success depends on the observance of certain general rules which may at any given moment be unpopular with the majority of the day. Hayek pleads for an acceptance of this vital truth which he accepts can only mean limitations on the power of majority governments.[77]

What had induced this damaging view of democratic government is what Hayek calls the 'constructivist positive superstition' – the view that governments, through their actions, can fundamentally change the world for the better. If government makes such claims, inevitably it becomes the target and then the creature of conglomerates of pressure groups as groups seek to advance their interests and competing parties seek their support. The result is an ever expanding and inevitably coercive web of government 'which threatens to strangle the growth of a civilisation which rests on individual freedom'.[78] When this constructivist interpretation of the order of society is combined with a mistaken understanding of the meaning of justice the spontaneous order is in acute danger. For it to survive men must reconcile themselves 'to the still strange fact that in a society of free men the highest authority must in normal times have no power of positive commands whatever'.[79] To get such a negative view of government accepted in a democracy characterised by party competition will, Hayek accepts, be extremely difficult but it is vital.

The heart of the argument can be summed up fairly easily. The pattern of democracy described above is a threat to the processes of spontaneous order which are the main source of general welfare. It is a threat to liberty because it extends the coercive actions of governments. It also gives undue power to particular interest groups of which the government bureaucracy is the most powerful. By putting an excessive burden on the sharing out function of government, social cohesion is strained. A particular group of people can be identified and blamed for particular economic and social outcomes.

These are the central issues which need explanation if the anti-collectivist attitude to the political system is to be appreciated. What the anti-collectivists want is limitations on the sphere of the political system. Because of this they want a decentralisation of power. At the same time, however, the state must be strong. General rules must be enforced. As Gamble puts it: 'The free economy requires a strong state'.[80] It is the sphere of activity not its power which must be limited.

As a corollary to their stress on the manifold virtues of the free market and their belief in freedom and individualism, anti-collectivists usually speak of 'the state' only to disparage it. It is a major boo word in the anti-collectivist vocabulary. 'Lift the curtain,' says Powell, 'and the state reveals itself as a little group of fallible men in Whitehall, making guesses about the future, influenced by political pressures and partisan prejudices.'[81] In the demonology of the British New Right 'the state' has an honoured place. 'It is "the state", writes Stuart Hall,

> which has overborrowed and overspent; fuelled inflation; fooled the people into thinking that there would always be more where the last handout came from; tried to assume the regulation of things like wages and prices which are best left to the hidden hand of market forces; above all interfered, meddled, intervened, instructed, directed – against the essence, the Genius of The British People.[82]

Role of government

'The central proposition', Bosanquet argues when summing up the social philosophy of the New Right, 'is that a major reduction in the role of government is both a necessary and a sufficient condition for progress.'[83] Although on the whole Hayek is prepared to accept a rather larger role for government than

Friedman, there is no doubt that the anti-collectivists have a general and abiding suspicion of government action – on three main grounds.

Firstly, anti-collectivists see government action as a threat to freedom. 'Every act of government intervention', Friedman asserts, 'limits the area of individual freedom directly and threatens the preservation of freedom indirectly.'[84] Secondly, they see government action as inherently inefficient and so as unlikely to achieve the desired objectives. It is inefficient because it depends ultimately on human wisdom rather than superior processes of the spontaneous order. Thirdly, government action is seen as socially disruptive in a variety of ways – in the expectations which it arouses, in the way the authority of government is weakened by its inevitable failure to make good its promises, and in the creation of new interest groups stimulated by more active government. Friedman sees a malevolent hand operating in the political sphere in contrast to the benevolent hand which operates in the economic arena. 'An individual', he suggests, 'who intends only to serve the public interest by fostering government intervention is led by an invisible hand to promote private interests which was no part of his intention.'[85] These private interests are in conflict with each other and therefore threatening to social order.

Anti-collectivists also seek to put government action in perspective. The great advances of civilisation, Friedman argues, have come from the initiative of individuals not from the actions of governments.[86] Hayek broadens the argument, urging that

> it is an error to believe that only actions which deliberately aim at common purposes serve common ends. The fact is rather that what the spontaneous order provides for us is more important for everyone, and therefore for the general welfare, than most of the particular services which the organisation of government can provide, excepting only the security provided by the enforcement of the rules of just conduct.[87]

In spite of their suspicion of government activity, anti-collectivists are agreed that there is an important, if narrowly circumscribed, role for government. Hayek is fiercely critical of the view that government activity should be limited to the maintenance of law and order. Such a view, he insists, 'cannot be justified by the principle of liberty. Only the coercive measures of government need to be strictly limited' and there is 'undeniably a wide field for the non-coercive activities of government'.[88] 'We need a strong state', says Mrs Thatcher, '. . . determined to maintain in good repair the frame which surrounds society. But the frame should not be so heavy or so elaborate as to dominate the whole picture.'[89]

What is that field? First and most important is the provision of the necessary framework for the efficient functioning of the spontaneous order. 'Competition can be made more effective and more beneficent', Hayek suggests, 'by certain activities of government than it would be without them.'[90] Most obviously, for example, a competitive economic system 'needs an intelligently designed and continuously adjusted legal framework'.[91] So there is a clear role for government both, in Sir Keith Joseph's words, 'as a maker of rules for men who want to fashion their lives for themselves'[92] and to ensure that the rules required for a spontaneous order are obeyed.

A second legitimate field of activity for government is in 'cases in which strictly voluntary exchange is either exceedingly costly or practically impossible. There are two general classes of such cases, monopoly and similar market imperfections and neighbourhood effects'.[93] Friedman accepts that in certain situations a monopoly may be necessary for reasons of efficiency and that a situation could arise when it was appropriate to entrust such a monopoly to government. Government intervention on grounds of neighbourhood effects arises 'when actions of individuals have effects on other individuals for which it is not feasible to charge or recompense them'.[94]

Hayek finds it 'unquestionable that in an advanced society government ought to use its power of raising funds by taxation to provide a number of services which for various reasons cannot be provided, or cannot be provided adequately by the market'.[95] He goes on to speak of 'the wide range of such wholly legitimate activities which, as the administrator of common resources, government may legitimately undertake'.[96] Hayek is also prepared to accept that there is 'some reason to believe' that with increases in general wealth and of the density of population the share of all needs that can be satisfied only by collective action will continue to grow.[97]

Thirdly, there is the paternalist role of government in relation to those designated by society as not capable of taking responsibility for themselves. Friedman's view is that 'there is no avoiding the need for some measure of paternalism'.[98] It is a duty 'susceptible of great abuse, yet it cannot be avoided'.[99] The risk of abuse lies in the expansion of the categories of individuals and groups regarded as not responsible and the threat this poses to freedom and industrial responsibility.

In Britain, criticism of the expanded role of government has been a central element in New Right arguments. It is a theme to which Mrs Thatcher has returned again and again stressing 'an imperative need to stop the growth of government and to re-establish just what the functions of government are'. She has stressed the damage done to the economy through over-government, the wounds to a sense of individual, family and community responsibility which result and the way in which, as government has expanded, it has become less effective and less efficient.[100] Reduction of the role of government was one of the central themes of Mrs Thatcher's first government – through exportation of responsibilities from central government to local government and from central government to private industry, through the privatisation of services, through stress on the role and responsibility of family and neighbourhood.

Attitudes to the welfare state

As might be anticipated from the values of the anti-collectivists, their faith in the spontaneous order of the market system, and their suspicion of government activity, their attitude to the welfare state is fundamentally hostile.

This is not to suggest that anti-collectivists deny government any role in welfare. 'It would be quite false', Barry has argued, 'to say that liberals in general and Hayek in particular are opposed to the idea of a Welfare State.'[101] Anti-collectivists, however, are apprehensive about such a role. They see welfare state policies as threatening or damaging to central social values and institutions – the family, work incentives, economic development, individual freedom, for example – and in general they are opposed to provision which is more than minimal.

Hayek has perhaps made most effort to define which welfare activities can be regarded as legitimate for government. Such activities, he has suggested, are entirely compatible with liberal principles so long as three conditions obtain – that government does not claim a monopoly, that resources are raised by taxation on uniform principles and taxation is not used as an instrument for income redistribution, and that the wants to be satisfied are collective wants of the community as a whole and not merely collective wants of particular groups.[102]

Hayek accepts that it is a responsibility of government to guarantee a social minimum. He speaks of the need for some such arrangement as 'unquestioned'.[103] When it becomes 'the recognised duty of the public to provide for the extreme needs of old age, unemployment, sickness etc.', Hayek sees it 'as an obvious corollary to compel them to insure (or otherwise provide) against those common hazards of life'.[104] Guaranteeing a basic minimum income, in Hayek's view, 'appears not only to be a wholly legitimate protection against a risk common to all, but a necessary part of the great society in which the individual no longer has specific claims on the members of the particular small group into which he was born'.[105] Minimal state provision may be unproblematic, but as Hayek sees it, 'a government dependent on public opinion, and particularly a democracy, will not be able to confine much attempts to supplement the market to the mitigation of the lot of the poorest . . . it is certain to be driven on by the principles implicit in the precedents it sets'.[106] A concern for a minimum leads on to a concern about inequality and the pursuit of the mirage of social justice. Anti-collectivists see such expansion as inevitable because of two factors – firstly, because of the nature of democratic government which leads to competition between parties for votes and so contributes to an expansion in the promises and activities of governments and, secondly, because of the pressures for expansion generated internally by welfare bureaucracies. To amateur and inexpert politicians the arguments they advance for expansion are compelling. State action leads, by its own inherent logic, therefore, to a situation which is quite unacceptable to anti-collectivists. Welfare state policies, if not tightly limited in a way which the anti-collectivists recognise as politically almost impossible, represent a dangerous shuffle down the road to egalitarianism and socialism.

When government moves beyond minimum provision anti-collectivist anxieties increase. It is possible to categorise their anxieties and objections under seven headings. The first and in some sense the major concern is the threat to freedom implicit in welfare state policies. Seldon puts it in extreme terms. 'The welfare state', he fulminates, 'has gradually changed from the expression of compassion to an instrument of political repression unequalled in British history and in other Western industrial societies.'[107]

What precisely is the basis of this threat to freedom? One element emphasised by Seldon is the way in which, *de facto*, the welfare state imposes maximum standards on people.[108] Having paid the taxes which finance collective welfare, most people cannot then afford to make private provision. They therefore have no real alternative but to accept the standard of service provided by the state. In Seldon's view 'the British welfare state has logically and ineluctably become the main instrument for the creation of equality by coercion'.[109]

Another blow to freedom inflicted by the welfare state is the way it allows or enables majorities to coerce minorities and individuals. Even if they might not wish to do so, minorities and individuals have to pay through taxation for particular services of a particular standard. Such services may be intended for their use but individuals might still prefer to do without them and spend their money in other ways. In a welfare state they cannot do this. The majority decides what shall be spent on particular goods and services. Minorities who object or who have other priorities cannot escape.

Freedom is also threatened by government monopolies in service provision and the lack of choice which results. Inevitably, too, public provision of services gives immense power to the bureaucrats and professionals who make judgments about need because, in Friedman's words, such services 'put some people in a position to decide what is good for other people. The effect is to instill in the one group a feeling of almost god-like power; in the other a feeling of childlike dependence.'[110]

Anti-collectivists are deeply pessimistic about the chances of genuine democratic control of government activities. 'It is sheer illusion to think', Hayek argues, 'that when certain needs of the citizen have become the exclusive concern of a single bureaucratic machine, democratic control of that machine can then effectively guard the liberty of the citizen'[111] in contrast to the dispersed power characteristic of the market.

A second anxiety which disturbs anti-collectivists is the effect of welfare state policies on government. A government committed to more than a minimum of welfare provision inevitably becomes a focus of pressure from a range of interests seeking action to redress grievances and injustices. In democracies, governments depend on support. Inevitably, therefore, governments seek to satisfy particular interests. They cease to be simply makers of general rules and umpires of the spontaneous order. In the process they all too easily become creatures of powerful interests or groups. 'Once we give licence to the politicians to interfere in the spontaneous order of the market for the benefit of particular groups', says Hayek, 'they cannot deny such concessions to any group on which their support depends.'[112] Governments become weakened and so less able to perform their most fundamental duty effectively – assisting the maintenance of the spontaneous order through the making of general rules.

A third broad area of criticism is that welfare state policies are destabilising to the economic and social system. We have already outlined the basis for the anti-collectivist anxiety about public expenditure (cf. p. 29). The argument that the welfare state contributes to the destabilising of the social system is based on ideas about the implications of the politicisation of issues of resource use and distribution. Welfare state policies feed the notion that these processes are susceptible to modification and alteration. Political pressure inevitably follows such a realisation. 'Social conflict is intensified by the welfare state', says Seldon, 'because it uses the political process to decide the use of resources, though "representative institutions" that are in practice controlled by *un*representatives who happen to be politically endowed.'[113]

A fourth, more specific charge against state welfare provision is that it is not responsive to individual and group needs because of the nature of such provision. A public service provides what officials, professionals and politicians *think* people need. Judgments are made not by consumers but by other people on their behalf. Anti-collectivists contrast this situation with a market system where consumers choose what they want from a range of goods and services provided by producers who stand or fall by their ability to provide the products that consumers want. If one believes, as do the anti-collectivists, that the consumer knows best, then 'the supply of goods and services, including medical care, should as nearly as possible be based upon individual preferences'.[114] That means a market system rather than publicly organised services.

A fifth charge levelled by the anti-collectivists is that state provision of welfare is fundamentally inefficient. Because bureaucratically provided services are less responsive to particular needs than market systems they will be less efficient at meeting those needs. The lack of competition in welfare provision will lead to ossification and a lack of experiment and innovation. Lees describes the absence of competition in the National Health Service as one of the service's most serious weaknesses. Because of the importance of experiment and innovation in the progress of health services, he regards medical care as 'one of the last commodities that should be monopolised by the state'.[115] Writing of pension provision Friedman argues that 'individual freedom to choose, and competition of private enterprises for custom would provide improvements in the kind of contracts available and foster variety and diversity to meet individual need'.[116]

Friedman argues that the very nature of welfare spending makes for inefficiency. All welfare spending falls into two categories of expenditure – spending someone else's money on yourself which makes for extravagance and a lack of concern to keep costs down, and spending someone else's money on a third person which again leads to a lack of concern for economy and, in addition, provides a lack of incentive to obtain for the third party the service he will value most highly. 'These characteristics of welfare spending', in Friedman's view, 'are the main source of their defects.'[117] Public services lack the two basic disciplines of the market – close concern with costs and sensitivity to consumer preferences. Inefficiency and ineffectiveness are therefore inevitable.

Another aspect of the inefficiency attacked by the anti-collectivists is the way in which the benefits of welfare programmes accrue only to a limited extent to those to whom they are directed. This is because of the strength of forces making for their misdirection. Interest groups press for services and legislation for their particular benefit – and the more successful groups are seldom groups of the poorest and the most needy. Universal, free services are often of most benefit to middle- and upper-income groups. The weaker and poorer members of society are as disadvantaged in the political market as in the economic market. In addition a major slice of all welfare programmes goes to those who staff and administer the programmes.[118]

There are two other related points in the charge of inefficiency. The first is that free services lead either to an excessive consumption of resources or to unsatisfactory and unacceptable attempts by bureaucrats to assess the validity of claims and pronounce on the relative importance of needs. This excess demand exacerbates another fundamental difficulty for state welfare services – raising the revenue required. The problem is a simple one – people's reluctance to pay taxes for services they do not or may not need when they could be using their money to meet real, current needs. Anti-collectivists see as fundamental the problem that the state will never be able to raise sufficient revenue to provide services equivalent in quality to those which would be supplied by the market system.[119]

The sixth charge which is levelled by anti-collectivists is that the welfare state has led to the neglect of other sources and systems of welfare and inhibited and hindered their development. They would see three sources and systems of welfare as more important than state services – the family, the voluntary sector and the market. They argue that all three have been damaged by the welfare state.

In the past, Friedman argues, 'Children helped their parents out of love and duty. They now contribute to the support of someone else's parents out of compulsion and fear. The earlier transfers strengthened the bonds of the family; the compulsory transfers weaken them.'[120] The same thesis is implicit in Mrs Thatcher's argument that 'if we are to sustain, let alone extend, the level and standard of care in the community, we must first try to put responsibility back where it belongs: with the family and with the people themselves'.[121]

Seldon has argued strongly that when assessing the supposed achievements of the welfare state we must not forget the array of welfare services it prevented from developing.[122] Specifically, he argues that

> The NHS has done the health of the people a 'dis-service' because it has prevented the development of more spontaneous, organic, local voluntary and *sensitive* medical services that would have grown up as incomes rose and medical science and technology advanced. If it were not for the *politically*-controlled NHS we should have seen new forms of medical organisation and financing that better reflected *consumer* preferences, requirements and circumstances.[123]

The primacy of family, voluntary and market services – the supposedly 'natural' sources of welfare – has been a continuing theme in New Right apologetics in Britain. As Patrick Jenkin put it when Secretary of State for Social Services, 'The Social services departments should seek to meet directly only those needs which others cannot or will not meet . . . Their task is to act as a safety net, the final protector for people for whom there is no other, not at a first port of call.'[124] 'I believe', Mrs Thatcher told the National Conference of the Women's Royal Voluntary Service, 'that the voluntary movement is at the heart of all our social welfare provision, that the statutory services are the supportive ones, underpinning where necessary, filling the gaps and helping the helpless.'[125]

The last charge we need to consider is the accusation that the welfare state is damaging to people. We have seen already the accusation that it is damaging to the family and family responsibility. There are also the more specific charges that public provision induces dependency, demoralisation, and irresponsibility and saps initiative, self-reliance and other desirable

Victorian values and virtues. The capacity of the beneficiaries of welfare programmes for independence and for making their own decisions, Friedman asserts, 'atrophies through disuse'. The end result of the whole miserable business is 'to rot the moral fabric that holds a decent society together'.[126]

It remains to say a little about anti-collectivist attitudes to individual social services.

Anti-collectivists agree that the state has a duty to relieve poverty but see that as the limit of state responsibility. They therefore favour minimum benefits based on means tests. Public schemes aimed at income maintenance in sickness, old age or unemployment are an illegitimate extension of this duty. So too are benefits paid to all irrespective of need and schemes aimed at egalitarian redistribution.

Anti-collectivists condemn the insurance principle as fraudulent, as a mechanism used to introduce backdoor socialism and as a way of imposing higher rates of taxation without proper debate. In practice, they argue, contributions are a tax on employment. They therefore discourage employers from hiring workers and increase unemployment. Government schemes of social insurance are virtual monopolies with all that means for inflexibility and inefficiency. This means that they are an assault on freedom. They both deprive us 'of control over a sizeable fraction of our income'[127] and give us no choice over the type and level of benefits we wish to purchase.

Friedman's summary of the blessings which would accrue from a winding down of public social security provision is comprehensive. In his view it

would eliminate its present effect of discouraging employment and so would mean a larger national income currently. It would add to personal saving and so lead to a higher rate of capital formation and a more rapid rate of growth of income. It would stimulate the development and expansion of private pension schemes and so add to the security of many workers.[128]

In housing, there is general agreement among anti-collectivists that government intervention has worsened rather than improved the situation. Rent control and subsidy are the two chief villains. In Powell's words – and Hayek makes the same point – 'You have only to reduce the price of anything below the point at which current supply and demand balance to create shortages in the present and repress production in the future.'[129] Hayek and

Friedman also stress the individually and socially damaging effects of public housing. As Hayek puts it, people 'become subject to arbitrary decisions of authority in their daily affairs and accustomed to looking for permission and direction in the main decisions of their lives'.[130] Anti-collectivist policy will therefore be directed to the rejuvenation of the private market in housing through the abolition of rent control and subsidy and the running down of the public sector.

Anti-collectivists accept the case for state provision of a compulsory minimum of education because it is better for all if all are educated and because a minimum of education is a necessary precondition for democratic government. The basis for anti-collectivists' anxiety about the state's role in provision beyond a minimum is that the major beneficiary is the individual and not society. There is therefore no case for state subsidies to vocational education which increase the earning power of the recipient. On the other hand, there may be a case for subsidies to non-vocational education because such education benefits the community at large as much, if not more, than the recipients.

The most distinctive contribution which the anti-collectivists have made to the debate about education provision is their advocacy of educational vouchers to be cashed by parents at government-approved schools of their choice. The argument for vouchers is based on the belief that the recreation of a market situation in education – schools supplying and parents buying – will increase parental choice, raise standards through competition between schools and reduce inequality.[131]

Anti-collectivists are firmly opposed to the public provision of free health care. They see health care as a commodity, no different in essence from other goods and services which the market system supplies more efficiently than any other mechanism. By definition, a publicly provided service will be inferior because of people's reluctance to pay the taxes to finance it; it will be inefficient because not stimulated by competition; it will offer individuals little or no choice; it will be cluttered by bureaucracy. However prodigal the public provision, resources will still have to be rationed and rationing in public services is less fair than rationing by price. In the British National Health Service, rationing, according to Seldon, is 'by influence and bully power'.[132]

The anti-collectivists' attitudes to individual services can generally be predicted from their values, their attitudes to society and the state and their views on the proper role of government. Their concern for freedom predisposes them against public provision. So too does their confidence in the superiority of market provision in terms of quality, price, efficiency of production, flexibility of response to need and demand. Their commitment to freedom and the market underpins their apprehensions about any extension of the range of government activity.

Understandably, the anti-collectivists are depressed that misconceived notions about the beneficence and superiority of state welfare provision have gained such a hold in so many countries. But history, they are confident, is on their side. Seldon is confident that the move from the welfare state to welfare provided primarily by the market is just round the corner. Market forces are stronger than political power just as good is ultimately stronger than evil.

Seldon's sources of hope are numerous. Rising incomes, he believes, will mean people will want more responsive services than the state can supply. The improved position of women in society will give a boost to provision through the market because women have a clearer appreciation of the advantages of competition from their experience of its benevolent impact on their supermarket shopping. The inequities of the welfare state will become more apparent. Technical innovation will expand to provide substitutes for state services. There will be an increasing rejection by minority groups of standardised state services. Increased tax evasion and avoidance will make the financing of acceptable levels of services increasingly problematic.[133] With such grounds of hope the anti-collectivists wait confidently for the collapse of the walls of the welfare state.

3

The reluctant collectivists

The reluctant collectivists are a clear if ill-defined group. They are distinct from the anti-collectivists in their lack of faith in an unregulated free market system. They believe in the necessity and beneficent possibilities of a government managed economy. At the same time, they distinguish themselves from the Fabians by their enthusiastic approval for private enterprise, their reluctant acceptance of government action and their rejection of enthusiastically egalitarian policies. In so far as they are radical, they are radicals to protect and conserve, not to change. 'The architects of the Keynesian revolution', says Heald, 'were not political or social revolutionaries; rather, as far-sighted members of the old social order, they saw how much else widespread misery and unemployment put at risk.'[1]

Social values

In many respects the values of the reluctant collectivists are similar to those of the anti-collectivists. Both groups emphasise their belief in liberty, individualism and in competitive private enterprise. The reluctants, however, hold fewer absolute values. Their values tend to be conditional and to be qualified by their intellectual pragmatism.

Their pragmatism is the product of the conviction that capitalism is not self-regulating. They continue to believe that it is the best economic system, but they believe that to function

44

efficiently and fairly it requires judicious regulation and control. Its faults are serious, but they can be corrected. The beginning of wisdom, as they see it, is to study how the economic system actually works rather than how it should work according to abstract theory or how we would prefer it to work. 'It may well be that the classical theory represents the way in which we should like our economy to behave', Keynes wrote. 'But to assume that it actually does so is to assume our difficulties away.'[2] The 'key fact' about Keynes, Gilmour suggests, was his pragmatic approach. 'He saw that unemployment was an intolerable evil. He refused to accept that it was an inevitable one or that the problem would solve itself; and he proposed a remedy. Only later did he perfect his theory.'[3] Keynes repudiated the British economic tradition of abstract theorising which is a basic element in the anti-collectivist approach.

Their pragmatism leads the reluctants to the view that the nature and limits of state action cannot be settled on abstract grounds of principle, but must be determined on their merits in specific cases. 'There can be no unchanging rules for either the method or the extent of government intervention', Gilmour argues. 'Both will be determined by circumstances.'[4]

Beveridge always argued that there was no single way of achieving full employment. The best approach lay in 'a selective combination of methods: we need various types of general control . . . we need probably public monopoly ownership in certain fields, private enterprise subject to public control in other fields, private enterprise free of any save the general controls in yet other fields'.[5]

This approach fits well with how Harris summarises Beveridge's attitude towards socialism. 'He insisted', she writes, 'that socialism was a technique rather than a principle and a question of means rather than ends; it should be involved on a pragmatic basis when other methods were found wanting, it should be pursued where it works successfully and abandoned where it failed.'[6]

Galbraith's position is similar and leads him to the view that 'no natural superiority can be assumed either for the market or for planning . . . the error is in basing action on generalisation'.[7] The choice between private and public enterprise is therefore pragmatic rather than ideological – what will work best in a particular situation. In Galbraith's view the larger role for the state in economic and social affairs – what he calls 'the new socialism' – 'is not ideological; it is compelled by circumstances'.[8]

This pragmatism is underpinned by a strong humanism. It was

concern about the human implications of capitalism which led Keynes, Beveridge, Macmillan and Galbraith, in their different periods, and for very different reasons, to explore the nature of an economic system which seemed so hurtful to so many. Concern about unemployment was the inspiration of Keynes's major work. 'His basic view of life', says Joan Robinson, 'was aesthetic rather than political. He hated unemployment because it was stupid and poverty because it was ugly.'[9] Moggridge writes of 'Keynes' passionate concern for the world and its ills'.[10] Though he had many typically Conservative characteristics, his concern about social ills and his sensitivity to suffering led him to question the conventional economic orthodoxies. Beveridge's fundamental humanism comes out most clearly in his definition of full employment. It means, he said, that there will always be more vacant jobs than there are men without work, that the labour market should be a seller's market rather than a buyer's market. The buyer who has difficulty in purchasing labour suffers inconvenience or some reduction in his profits, whereas the seller who can find no market for his labour is told, in effect, that he is of no use. 'The first difficulty causes annoyance or loss. The other is a personal catastrophe.'[11] In Beveridge's eyes, the greatest evil of unemployment was not the loss of additional material wealth involved, but the fact that 'unemployment makes men seem useless, not wanted, without a country'.[12] Keynes and Beveridge would both have accepted Galbraith's judgment that society's highest task is 'to reflect on its pursuit of happiness and harmony and its success in expelling pain, tension, sorrow, and the ubiquitous curse of ignorance'.[13]

Freedom is a fundamental value for the reluctants. After first reading *The Road to Serfdom*, Keynes wrote to Hayek that: 'Morally and philosophically I find myself in agreement with virtually the whole of it, and not only in agreement with it, but in a deeply moved agreement.'[14] He went on, however, to disassociate himself from Hayek's views on planning. Beveridge stressed on many occasions that his aim was full employment in a free society. He regarded certain liberties as essential – freedom of worship, speech, writing, study and teaching, freedom of assembly and association for political or other purposes, freedom in choice of occupation and freedom in the management of a personal income.[15] They were 'more precious than full employment itself'.[16] At the end of the day, however, Beveridge's approach to questions of freedom was essentially pragmatic – some freedoms were more important than others and some restrictions on freedom more acceptable in pursuit of other goals.

Beveridge also saw what the anti-collectivists tend to forget or ignore, that 'Liberty means more than freedom from the arbitrary power of governments. It means freedom from economic servitude to Want and Squalor and other social evils.'[17] As Harold Macmillan put it: 'It is only in so far as poverty is abolished that freedom is increased.'[18]

The reluctant collectivists lay great stress on individualism, private enterprise and self-help. These beliefs are what underlie their preference for capitalism over other forms of economic organisation. Keynes speaks of 'the traditional advantages of individualism' and proceeds to describe them.[19]

> They are partly advantages of efficiency – the advantages of decentralisation and of the self-interest. . . . But above all, individualism, if it can be purged of its defects and its abuses, is the best safeguard of personal liberty in the sense that, compared with any other system, it greatly widens the field for the exercise of personal choice. It is also the best safeguard of the variety of life, which emerges precisely from this extended field of personal choice, or the loss of which is the greater of all the losses of the homogeneous or totalitarian state.

Individualism and private enterprise were important to Keynes for two other reasons – as vital sources of individual innovation and initiative – 'New forms and modes spring from the fruitful minds of individuals', as he put it.[20]

Beveridge shared Keynes's views. 'The State', he wrote, 'is or can be master of money, but in a free society it is master of very little else. The making of a good society depends not on the State but on the citizens acting individually or in free association with one another.'[21] Beveridge's proposals to secure and maintain full employment had the aim, as he put it, 'of keeping private enterprise as servant not as master'.[22]

In their attitude to equality and inequality the reluctant collectivists separate themselves very clearly from both the Fabian socialists and the Marxists. They are committed defenders of inequality for a range of reasons. Beveridge saw differences of reward as vital to a free and efficient labour market. 'Economic rewards for effort and economic punishment for failure of effort', he concluded, 'are the alternative to the chain gang.'[23] Keynes argued the social or cultural case for inequality. In his view, says Harrod, 'the first claim upon the national dividend was to furnish these few, who were capable of "passionate perception", with the ingredients of what modern civilisation can provide by way of a "good life".'[24] He also believed that 'there are valuable human activities which require the motive of money making and the environment of private wealth ownership for their full function'.[25]

Keynes did, however, conclude in *The General Theory* that certain historic justifications for inequality were out of date. The growth of wealth, he wrote, 'so far from being dependent on the abstinence of the rich, as is commonly supposed, is more likely to be impeded by it. One of the chief social justifications of greater inequality of wealth, whether acquired or inherited is, therefore, removed'.[26] If growth depends on spending rather than saving, inequality can be dysfunctional, greater equality more functional.

Gilmour makes a three-pronged attack on egalitarianism and so an implicit defence of inequality. He sees egalitarianism as economically disastrous because

> a competitive economy cannot work well if adequate rewards are withheld from those who do difficult and responsible jobs, from those who are prepared to take risks with their money, and from those who have to undergo long training before they can gain the necessary qualifications to practise their profession or occupation.[27]

Egalitarianism also, he believes, 'weakens rather than strengthens social cohesion' and must be regarded as a threat to freedom because of the policies required for its implementation.[28]

On the other hand, the reluctant collectivist position on equality and inequality is significantly different from that of the anti-collectivists. They are not egalitarians but they think that inequalities should and could be reduced. Gilmour contrasts what he regards as the Conservative position on equality – a reluctant collectivist stance – with Hayek's position, pointing out that although Conservatives do not favour the imposition of economic equality they can, nevertheless, easily conceive of a distribution of income which would be intolerable and would require adjustment – for example, through progressive taxation. Anti-collectivists, in contrast, regard any government measures to modify the pattern of distribution delivered by the market as unacceptable.[29]

Beveridge also pressed a moral and economic case for greater equality. The moral argument, as he saw it, is that the same amount of wealth will yield more happiness if it is distributed widely than if it is concentrated. The economic case – made against a background of depression – is that a more equal distribution of wealth and income will increase aggregate demand and so contribute to the goal of full employment.

All the reluctant collectivists, however, would see a concern about poverty as distinct from and more important than the search for equality. That is their prior concern.

Society and the state

The reluctant collectivists' analysis of society concentrates almost entirely on the economic system. Being basically conservative, they accept the social and political order as given. They have little to say about class and only Galbraith is seriously concerned with questions of power.

As regards societal organisation the reluctants see society as characterised by consensus rather than conflict. They would, however, lay less stress than the anti-collectivists on the unifying power of the market system. Beveridge and Gilmour are both clearly apprehensive about how an unregulated market system could be socially divisive and a source of protest and conflict. They do not, however, see class or group differences as irreconcilable but rather see economic and social developments as contributing to a reduction in social tension.

Galbraith argues that economic growth has led, in the USA, to a decline in concern with the patterns of income distribution. Economic growth, he suggests, functions as the 'solvent of the tensions once associated with inequality' for three reasons. It increases social mobility so reducing concern about inequality. It has led to a decline in conspicuous consumption by the very rich and so to less interest in their position and the inequalities they represent. Thirdly, economic growth has fostered a greater social pluralism. The prestige of the merely rich has been eroded by the countervailing prestige of politicians, technocrats, managers, TV idols, and so on.[30]

The central element in the reluctant collectivist view of the economic system is the sharp critique of unregulated capitalism which is presented. This needs, however, to be set against a basic confidence that the central mechanisms of capitalism – competition, private enterprise, the profit motive, the price system and the free market – can, when duly modified and regulated, form the best basis for economic activity. David Owen, indeed, argues that economic growth is only possible within the framework of the mixed economy.[31] Pure capitalism and pure socialism offer no hope. William Rodgers argues in similar terms stressing both 'the unacceptable characteristics of a "free market" and the necessity to harness the basic market elements of profits, competition and markets if the economy is to function efficiently'.[32] Owen sees 'no incompatibility between working towards greater efficiency, through free competitive markets and greater equality through a redistributive social reform policy'.[33]

The reluctant collectivists' critique of capitalism can be explored under four main headings – capitalism is not self-regulating; it is wasteful and inefficient and misallocates resources; it will not of itself abolish injustice and poverty; it creates conditions which can be threatening to political stability.

The doctrine of a self-regulating economic system was a very comfortable one. It included two essential articles – that regulatory action by the state was necessary neither on economic nor political grounds. State action on economic grounds was unnecessary because, according to Say's Law of Markets, production automatically created its own sufficient demand. 'Whether or not a person accepted Say's Law', says Galbraith, 'was, until the 1930s, the prime test by which economists were distinguished from crackpots.'[34]

A self-regulating capitalism raised no political problems either. The consumer was sovereign. Competition ensured that he remained the ultimate authority. Neither consumers nor workers could be exploited because they would simply take their custom or their labour elsewhere. As Galbraith puts it, 'if choice by the public is the source of power, the organisations that comprise the economic system cannot have power. They are merely instruments in the ultimate service of that choice'.[35] The economic system is thus democratised. Ultimate power in economic as well as political affairs rests with the individual. 'The public through the consumer being already in charge, the public through the government need not and should not intervene.'[36]

Keynes was a fierce critic of *laissez-faire*. 'It is not true', he wrote, 'that individuals possess a prescriptive "natural liberty" in their economic activities. There is no compact conferring perpetual rights on those who Have or those who Acquire. The world is not so governed from above that private and social interest always coincide.'[37] But Keynes's great achievement was to destroy the notion of a self-regulating economic system and provide the theoretical underpinning for a new economics. He demonstrated that the inter-war depression was in effect a refutation of Say's Law and showed that there was no technical reason why demand and production should be in balance. Such an analysis, says Stewart, was 'dramatic' and 'imperative', 'dramatic because it stood existing economic theory on its head, imperative because it implied the need for government action of a kind, and on a scale never before contemplated'.[38]

Keynes saw the key weakness of the market economy as deficiency of demand. Beveridge's view was that the demand for labour was not merely inadequate but misdirected. He therefore wanted government action on three lines – to maintain total outlay at all times; to control the location of industry and direct it to regions where the demand for labour was inadequate; and to secure the organised mobility of labour to meet industry's unmet need.[39]

Keynes's thinking was about the failure of the unregulated economy to ensure sufficient demand to avoid depression and unemployment. Beveridge had the same preoccupation. Galbraith takes the discussion of the non-self-regulating economy and applies it to the affluent capitalism which is the essential product and achievement of the Keynesian revolution. Given the application of Keynesian techniques of economic management and the achievement of near full employment, Galbraith sees the resulting system as in desperate need of government control and regulation. Keynes hoped that within a proper framework of government economic policy the economic system could again become self-regulating. Galbraith shows that this dream has not come true. Owen and Rodgers believe that market forces can be harnessed by government to give the best of all worlds.

The main thesis which Galbraith has developed so powerfully is that technological development increases industry's need for state help. Industry needs highly trained manpower and it relies on the state to supply it. It needs investment funds for exciting but uncertain projects. The development of new products requires a heavy advance commitment of money, time and manpower. Industry must be able to be confident that there will, in the end, be a market for the product. In this situation, 'The regulation of aggregate demand . . . is an organic requirement of the industrial system.'[40]

In an affluent society, state regulation of demand is more necessary than in a poorer society because, with affluence, saving and spending become much more matters for individual and corporate choice and decision. 'In consequence', Galbraith argues, 'in a community of high well-being, spending and hence demand are less reliable than in a poor one. They lose their reliability precisely when high costs and the long period of gestation imposed by modern technology require greater certainty of markets'.[41] The real enemy of the market, therefore, is not socialism but advanced technology.[42]

Galbraith further develops this thesis arguing that in the absence of state intervention the planning system (i.e. the giant corporations) is inherently unstable, subject to recession and depression which are not self-limiting as in simpler economies, but which can become cumulative.[43] In simpler economies there are natural mechanisms which operate to stop the downward movement of economic activity from becoming cumulative. In the planning system these do not operate. Prices do not fall because they are controlled by the firm; wages cannot be reduced because of the strength of the trade unions.

Galbraith has emphasised one further way in which advanced capitalism is not self-regulating – its inability to control inflation. Keynes had foreseen the problem as early as 1944. 'I do not doubt', he wrote then, 'that a serious problem will arise when we have a combination of collective bargaining and full employment.' In his view it was 'a political rather than an economic problem'.[44] Beveridge anticipated the problem too but with the advantage of thirty years' experience of inflation; Galbraith has sharpened the analysis. The key factor which makes inflation 'an organic feature of the industrial system',[45] is that prices are now determined not by the market but by the firm. This means that the individual firm will not put up more than a token resistance to wage demands because it can finance them by raising prices. There is no body which can supply general restraint except the state. So there is no alternative to state action.[46]

Keynes and Beveridge seem to be making different criticisms of capitalism from Galbraith. In fact, all are concerned to stress capitalism's inability to achieve self-regulation and to suggest how public action can make good this failing without destroying the system. What Harrod said of Keynes could be applied to Beveridge and Galbraith as well. 'His lifelong effort to understand what is wrong with the machine', he wrote, 'implies that he wanted us to continue to use the machine, implies, in fact, that he was at bottom an individualist.'[47]

The second major charge which the reluctant collectivists bring against unregulated capitalism is that it is wasteful and inefficient and leads to an unsatisfactory allocation of resources. Keynes and Beveridge were both appalled by the waste involved in the inter-war depression. 'Failure to use our productive powers', Beveridge stressed, 'is the source of an interminable succession of evils.'[48] As he argued in his social insurance plan, want could have been abolished in the inter-war years had government so willed.[49] Keynes expressed his similar 'profound conviction that the Economic Problem, as one may call it for short, the problem of want and poverty and the economic struggle between classes and nations, is nothing but a frightful muddle, a transitory and an unnecessary muddle'.[50]

For Keynes and Beveridge the problem was an economy which was failing to use its productive capacity to the full. For Galbraith, the problem was the use to which a successful economic system was putting its productive capacities. He criticised the 'ubiquitous' and 'obtrusive' contrast between private affluence and public squalor which he saw as inherent in the advanced capitalist economy. Such a contrast, he argued, was not only offensive, it was also dangerous. 'An austere community is free from temptation. It can be austere in its public services. Not so a rich one.'[51] If it is austere, problems of crime, vandalism, violence and drug abuse are more likely to proliferate.

In his later writings, Galbraith locates the reasons for this social imbalance firmly in the nature of capitalism. Not all public services, he realised, were deprived of resources. 'This deprivation was great where public needs were involved, non-existent where powerful industry pressed its requirements on the State.'[52] Defence, research and technological developments, highways and air traffic management were not neglected because they were demanded by powerful voices. But the care of the ill, the old, the physically and mentally handicapped, the provision of recreational facilities, the problem of poverty were urged by no powerful voices. They were thus neglected.[53]

Because of their values, the waste and patterns of allocation of an unregulated capitalism are intolerable to the reluctant collectivists. They do not regard these ills as inevitable but as susceptible to control and elimination by due and proper regulation.

The third charge levelled at capitalism by the reluctant collectivists is that economic development will not, as a natural and inevitable outcome of rising general prosperity, abolish poverty and injustice. Beveridge saw this and emphasised its importance, pointing out that the growing general prosperity and rising real wage levels between 1900 and 1939 had diminished want, but still left a sizeable problem. 'The moral', he concluded, 'is that new measures to spread prosperity are needed.'[54]

Galbraith pointed out the same truth, the argument strengthened by the passing of time and faster growth. Increasing aggregated output, he emphasised, 'leaves a self-perpetuating margin of poverty at the very base of the income pyramid'.[55] He urged that an income necessary for decency and comfort should be secured for all 'as a normal function of the society'.[56] He sees the failure of economic growth to abolish poverty as one aspect of the many sided social imbalance inherent in the advanced capitalist economy. By its very nature it generates and perpetuates inequality and poverty.

The fourth charge which the reluctant collectivists level at capitalism is that sectional interests come to be equated with the public interest so creating conditions threatening to political stability. The sectional interests which dominate in America are those of the planning system. To survive and flourish, advanced capitalism must cultivate an ethos which encourages people to acquire and consume its products. Production, therefore, becomes a god. Industry has the key to the good life if not to the gates of heaven. When industry needs government help, it gets it, because what serves industry and production serves the national interest. The locus of power in the planning system is the technostructure. It is made up of the most prestigious, affluent and articulate members of the community. Their views on public policy, therefore, command immense and solemn respect.

> What serves the technostructure – the protection of its autonomy of decision, the promotion of economic growth, the stabilisation of aggregate demand, the acceptance of its claim to superior income, the provision of qualified manpower, the government services and investment that it requires, the other requisites of success – IS the public interest.[57]

The dominance of the planning system and the establishment of its interest as the public interest help to explain many of the inefficiencies, injustices and other blots on the capitalist copybook. Galbraith sees this colonisation of the state as a major flaw and weakness in advanced capitalism as an economic and political system, and as a major obstacle to be overcome if capitalism is to be reformed.

Gilmour sums up the argument about the dangers of the system Galbraith describes.

> A free state will not survive unless its people feel loyalty to it. And they will not feel loyalty unless they gain from the state protection and other benefits. Lectures on the ultimate beneficence of competition and on the dangers of interfering with market forces will not satisfy people who are in trouble. If

the state is not interested in them, why should they be interested in the state?

In the Conservative view, therefore, economic liberalism, *à la* Professor Hayek, because of its starkness and its failure to create a sense of community, is not a safeguard of political freedom but a threat to it.[58]

Shirley Williams argues the same kind of case from a different position on the reluctant collectivist continuum. 'The welfare state', she says, 'has been a crucial element in maintaining the political stability of the Western world in the turbulent post-war years.'[59]

In spite of these various criticisms, what is required, in the view of the reluctant collectivists, is not that capitalism be superseded, but that it be regulated and reformed. Keynes did not believe that 'there is any economic improvement for which revolution is a necessary instrument'.[60] Beveridge took the same view. 'The necessity of socialism, in the sense of nationalisation of the means of production, distribution and exchange, in order to secure full employment', he wrote, 'has not yet been demonstrated.'[61] If, however, it was shown that the abolition of private enterprise was necessary to achieve full employment 'this would have to be undertaken'.[62]

Keynes devoted most of his life to criticising the workings of the capitalist system and yet he remained a firm supporter of its fundamental principles. He concluded his fierce attack *The End of Laissez-Faire* with the reflection that 'capitalism, wisely managed, can probably be made more efficient for attaining economic ends than any alternative system yet in sight' although 'it is in many ways extremely objectionable'.[63] Seymour Harris concluded that 'Keynes' mission in life was to save capitalism, not destroy it'.[64]

Beveridge similarly stressed the non-political nature of his proposals both for social insurance and for securing full employment. They were, he insisted, neither socialism nor capitalism. 'A conscious control of the economic system at the highest level', he insisted, is '. . . required in any modern society.'[65]

Keynes and Beveridge were concerned with the capitalism of the Depression, Galbraith with the capitalism of the affluent society. Their attitudes, however, are remarkably similar. In his early writings, Galbraith could see 'no administratively acceptable alternative to the decision-making mechanism of capitalism'.[66] Public ownership would, in comparison, be clumsy and unresponsive, impracticable in the complex economic system of advanced industrial society. In his later writings, Galbraith is increasingly critical of many features of capitalism and he has come to believe that for some tasks capitalism is unsatisfactory. It is, for example, 'seriously incompetent in providing the things and services that cities most require . . . the modern city is, by its nature, a socialist enterprise'.[67] Such areas and services must be removed from the capitalist system and governed collectively.

But apart from the pragmatic, un-ideological New Socialism of necessity, Galbraith seems to continue to see capitalism as the main system of production and distribution. It is to be regarded as normal except when it fails, and then we should be brisk and businesslike, though a shade regretful, and accept socialism as a necessary and wholly normal feature of the system.

The way in which the faults, weaknesses and ills of capitalism are analysed is an important factor in the subsequent proposals. The reluctant collectivists are led by their analysis to the view that all can be made good through government action. Galbraith is led by his analysis to the most radical proposals but, although again and again he describes the ills of capitalism as 'systemic' (one of his favourite words), he nevertheless clings to the belief that 'systemic', 'inherent', 'organic' ills can be relieved without changes which would destroy or supersede the basic mechanisms of capitalism. In brief, Galbraith and the other reluctant collectivists are harshly critical of capitalism because they want to reform it. They want to pick out its weaknesses and failings so that they can be remedied. It is criticism for reform not destruction.

How do reluctant collectivists see the political system and the state? Essentially they occupy a position midway between that of the anti-collectivists and the Fabians, between a fundamental anxiety about state action and a fundamental enthusiasm for it. They are democrats but with some slight or considerable anxieties about the ability of majority governments to avoid becoming the creatures of interest groups. They vary too in their attitude to bureaucracy – from enthusiasm for the civil servant as the genuine apostle of the national interest and the public good, to apprehension that bureaucrats have usurped the power of politicians.[68] Essentially, however, their anxieties about the political system are minor and technical rather than substantial.

The reluctant collectivists spend little time on what the state is or how it operates. Implied in their writings, however, is the idea that the state is identical to the central government and is capable of independent, impartial action for the good of all. Sweezy talks of

'Keynes' habit of treating the State as a *deus ex machina* to be invoked whenever his human actors, behaving according to the rules of the capitalist game, get themselves into a dilemma from which there is apparently no escape'.[69] There is no sense in which either Keynes or Beveridge see the state as the focus of a range of conflicting interests. They see it as able to stand in an independent role of judgment on the functioning of the economic system, the performance of private enterprise, and the distribution of the national income.

Harris writes of Beveridge's 'highly optimistic view of the nature of the state and of its identification with the interests of the whole of society'.[70] Gilmour has no doubts that the state can act to make good the defects of the market system and provide protection and benefits for citizens. It is not the creature of any particular interests in society. It can act independently. Of course, the state *can* be a threat to liberty, 'But a state kept within bounds is not an enemy.'[71] The state and the individual are wrongly perceived if seen as mutually antagonistic. Rather they are mutually dependent and mutually sustaining.[72]

Galbraith does not fully share this optimism. As already mentioned he is quite clear that the state is, in fact, the creature of the dominant economic interest, what he styles the planning system. It has been successful in identifying its interests as the public interest but state action is, in fact, geared to the very particular interests of the planning system rather than the general interest. Nevertheless, Galbraith believes that the state can be emancipated from this sectional embrace and be recaptured 'for public purpose'[73] by a demonstration of the divergence between the planning interest and the public interest and by the inculcation of a new, critical, public awareness.

The role of government

Reluctant collectivists believe that government can function as an independent body concerned for and equipped to further the interests of all members of society. On essentially pragmatic grounds they support government action on these lines. By 1924, Keynes had decided that *laissez-faire* must be abandoned, 'not from contempt of that good old doctrine but because whether we like it or not, the conditions for its success have disappeared'.[74]

Fifty years later Gilmour was arguing in precisely the same terms. 'Laissez-faire', he concluded, 'is not an option.'[75] This view was the basis of Galbraith's socialism of circumstances – that

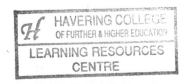

57

in area after area of economic and social life 'as a purely technical matter there is no alternative to public management'.[76]

Harris makes exactly the same point in her concluding discussion of Beveridge's views. 'Beveridge's ultimate commitment to a planned society', she writes, 'must be seen not as a reflection of his instinctive preferences, but as a reluctant recognition of what he believed to have become a practical necessity brought about by the fact that other methods of running complex industrial societies had manifestly failed.'[77]

The basic case for government intervention is pragmatic. The degree and extent of such action is also to be decided on pragmatic grounds. As Gilmour put it, 'there is no fixed frontier for the activities of the state'.[78] Economic and social aims and needs set those limits rather than abstract theories and beliefs and the government action required to achieve aims will vary from time to time according to circumstances. Human and social needs and aims are more important than abstract principles.

The second important respect in which the attitude of the reluctant collectivists differs from that of the Fabians is that, whereas Fabians see government essentially as an instrument for changing society, the reluctants are much more concerned with preserving a particular economic and social system. Government action is to enable what the reluctant collectivists see as the basic mechanisms of economic life to work more effectively.

The third point which needs to be made about the reluctant collectivists' attitude to the role of government is to emphasise elements of hesitancy about government intervention in the economy. Beveridge made it quite plain that he believed that the state should do whatever was required to secure full employment. At different times in his career this belief led him to urge state control of the means of production, at others to urge that state regulation of demand would be sufficient.[79] Other reluctant collectivists lack Beveridge's confidence in government. 'No Tory', wrote Gilmour, 'wants to substitute the judgements of civil servants or politicians as to the viability of investment projects for that of bankers and other professionals.'[80] Rodgers shared this anxiety. 'If there is one single step most likely to bring British industry to a final standstill', he concludes, 'it would be a decisive shift from decision in the boardroom to decisions in Westminster and Whitehall.'[81] Reluctant collectivists do not want government to control the economy, simply to provide treatment in those areas afflicted by malfunctioning.

So, although they believe that government has a positive part to play in economic and social life, the reluctant collectivists are keen to emphasise the limitations which they place on government activity. 'As a Radical', Beveridge said in 1945, 'I am not afraid of State control or public ownership where either of these is necessary to cure evils which cannot be cured without them, but my bias is against them not for them.'[82] 'The underlying principle of the Report', he wrote in *Full Employment*, 'is to propose for the State only those things which the State alone can do or which it can do better than any local authority or than private citizens either singly or in association, and to leave to these other agencies that which if they will they can do as well or better than the State.'[83]

A new strand in reluctant collectivist thinking which has emerged in the writings of the leaders of the Social Democratic Party is stress on the decentralisation of power. There is a reluctance to see power concentrated in Whitehall and Westminster. 'A true democracy', David Owen writes, 'will mean a progressive shift of power from Westminster out to the regions, to the county and town halls, to communities, neighbourhood, patients, tenants and parents.'[84] Such thinking clearly represents another dimension in traditional reluctant collectivist anxiety about concentrating power in the hands of government.

Despite their lingering anxieties and their stress on the limitations of government, the views of the reluctant collectivists implied a major expansion of government activity in a way which was qualitatively new. According to one reviewer of *Full Employment*:

> Too much of our economic thinking in the thirties awarded to the central government the dual function of running its own affairs and tinkering with the capitalist system in its spare time. Beveridge's thesis, on the other hand, is that the government, in running its own affairs, cannot ignore the effects of its actions on the capitalistic system, and must adjust its programs so that government and business jointly achieve full employment. The notion of the doctor prescribing for a sick patient is discarded in favour of the principle of partnership, with the qualification that the government is responsible if things go wrong.[85]

Beveridge was torn between his suspicion and dislike of government and his passionate determination to destroy the five Giants. His liberal principles led him to seek to stress the limitations which he believed should be applied to government action while, on the other hand, his passionate concern about

59

social ills led him at times to the view that many less essential liberties could rightly and reasonably be sacrificed to their abolition.

Like Beveridge, Keynes believed that government activity should be confined to achieving those results that could not be secured by uncoordinated individual effort.

> The most important Agenda of the State relate not to those activities which private individuals are already fulfilling but to the functions which fall outside the sphere of the individual, to those decisions which are made by no one if the State does not make them. The important thing for government is not to do things which individuals are doing already, and to do them a little better or a little worse, but to do those things which at present are not done at all.[86]

Over the years, Keynes became more tolerant of government intervention in social and economic life but this remained his basic position. To combine stress on the necessity and inevitability of government intervention and activity with stress on its limitation is, however, difficult. As Galbraith pointed out, Keynes 'though unobtrusively, opened the way for a large expansion of government services and activities'.[87]

Galbraith has a much wider view of the necessary sphere of state action than Keynes or Beveridge. In his view, the lines of economic and social development have greatly widened the area in which collectivist solutions must be applied. But it is still a reluctant and limited collectivism confined to issues where the normal solutions of private enterprise and the free market have been unsuccessful. It is a collectivism not of principle, but of necessity.

The reluctant collectivists, therefore, believe in limiting the role of government because of their belief in the ability of a free market system to regulate itself once a framework has been established, because of their belief in the natural superiority of private enterprise as a source of initiative and a bastion of liberty, and because of their suspicion that government action is a potential threat to freedom at the same time as they see it as necessary to freedom.

They are agreed on the ability and the duty of government to manage the economy so as to secure a level of aggregate demand which will ensure full employment. Keynes defended such action 'both as the only practicable means of avoiding the destruction of existing economic forms in their entirety and as the condition of the successful functioning of individual initiative'.[88] Beveridge similarly urged the responsibility of the state to maintain adequate total outlay and emphasised that this must be seen as a function of the state 'as definitely as it is now the function of the state to defend its citizens against attack from abroad or against robbery and violence at home'.[89] The state must assume this responsibility because 'no other authority or person has the requisite powers'.[90] The Second World War convinced Beveridge that there was no incompatibility between planning and democracy.

Keynes's basic concern was with economic management to provide a framework in which natural forces could operate. Beveridge is much more concerned with economic planning for social goals. He rejects certain approaches because they are socially unacceptable. The use of public investment to compensate for fluctuations in private investment is unacceptable because communal investment is too important to be kept on tap to fill gaps in private spending.[91] On similar grounds, Beveridge rejects a simple expansion of the private outlay approach as the whole answer. Such a policy is unlikely to be effective, he thinks, and it does nothing about the problem that there are many essential services which individuals either cannot get for themselves or can only get at excessive cost compared with the cost of collective provision.[92]

Keynes's work gave a new legitimacy to public expenditure. The traditional neo-classical view was that any expansion of public expenditure above what was directly necessary to the functioning of private enterprise was dangerous. This was because such investment absorbed resources which would otherwise have been profitably invested in industry. If, as Keynes argued, desired savings could exceed desired investment, then public expenditure was no longer necessarily at the expense of private investment, and so was not by definition bad and wasteful.[93]

Management of the economy to secure full employment has other implications for the role of state action. 'Adoption by the state of a price policy', Beveridge reckoned, 'is a natural and probably an inevitable consequence of a full employment policy.'[94] Galbraith has developed the argument and sees state regulation of wages and prices as the only way to combat the inflationary tendencies inherent in the fully employed corporate state.[95] Gilmour is equally convinced that an incomes policy is a necessary responsibility of government.[96] Owen argues that 'what must be developed is a policy for incomes, investment, prices, profit and productivity' – widening still further the sphere of government activity.[97] Such policies must, of course, have objectives – to preserve the existing patterns of distribution or to change them.

As regards planning for social welfare purposes, the reluctant collectivists see the responsibility of the government as starting from those social tasks considered to be necessary but only attainable through government action. 'There are vital things needing to be done to raise the standard of health and happiness in Britain', said Beveridge, 'which can only be done by common action.'[98] 'We cannot overcome social evils,' he urged elsewhere, 'without an extension of the responsibilities of the state.'[99] The inter-war economy, to which Beveridge looked back with such distaste, was characterised by two major ills – unused productive resources and crying social evils. Economic planning was aimed at the first, social planning at the second. The state must take the lead because it is the only body which can coordinate the onslaught on the giants blocking the road to reconstruction. They must be conquered because their domination means tyranny and misery which are bad in themselves and bad too because 'Misery generates hate'.

As depression returned to the world economy in the 1970s and 1980s, so concern developed again about the social and political stability of capitalist democracy. Gilmour lays great stress on citizen loyalty to the state as a factor in the maintenance of social order and stability. His argument is that if the state shows little manifest consideration for millions of its citizens they are unlikely to feel much affection and loyalty in return – this is a vital factor in his view of the proper role of government. 'The Tory emphasis on authority and loyalty', he insists, 'has always ruled out the night watchman state.'[100] Harold Macmillan, long before Gilmour, supported such a view arguing in *The Middle Way* that 'if capitalism had been conducted all along as if the theory of private enterprise were a matter of principle' and all state intervention had been resisted accordingly 'we should have had civil war long ago'.[101]

The welfare state

The reluctant collectivists accept the welfare state. They see it, however, as a mechanism for making good the failure of the market to control avoidable ills rather than an instrument for economic and social change or for promoting the good life. They accept the failure of the market to meet basic needs, the inability of the contemporary family to meet needs it supposedly met in the past and that economic growth will not, on its own, abolish poverty. Their values and a pragmatic concern for social order lead them to accept and espouse state welfare. As Gilmour puts it, speaking for one reluctant collectivist tradition, 'only liberal ideologues, not Conservatives, see something fundamentally wrong with the welfare state as such. State provision for welfare is fully in accordance with Conservative principles.'[102]

Keynes had little to say directly about what we think of as the welfare state, though he was clearly sympathetic towards an extension of welfare services.[103] Harrod says that the general philosophy of the Beveridge Report on Social Insurance accorded with Keynes's views and that he gave 'warm general support to the Beveridge proposals', though he persuaded Beveridge to reduce the commitment of the Exchequer in the early years.[104] It would have pleased Keynes as a humanitarian concerned for the abolition of avoidable social ills and it would have fitted his pleas for a redistribution of purchasing power to those most likely to spend.

For both Beveridge and Galbraith individual welfare was their ultimate concern. Subject to the preservation of essential liberties, Beveridge was prepared 'to use the powers of the state, so far as may be necessary without any limit whatever, in order to abolish the five giant evils'.[105] We must regard the five giants: Want, Disease, Ignorance, Squalor, and Idleness, he stressed, as common enemies, not as enemies with which each individual may seek a separate peace. 'That is the meaning of social conscience; that one should refuse to make a separate peace with social evil.'[106] Galbraith's whole critique of American capitalism is rooted and grounded in the belief that it does not serve individual welfare or the public interest. His aim is for a state concerned for welfare, the public interest and the good life – a welfare state.

Beveridge and Galbraith share a pragmatic approach to the role of the state in welfare. It is to abolish avoidable ills; the role is to be reactive rather than promotional; it is problem centred. Their concern is to supply what is not being supplied adequately by private enterprise, to abolish want whether due to low or interrupted incomes, and, in Galbraith's case, to supply the public services for which affluence has created a need and the lack of which actually causes poverty.

Beveridge's stress was on the achievement of a national minimum. He would have endorsed the sentiments of his former political master – Winston Churchill – that 'We want to draw a line below which we will not allow persons to live and labour, yet above which they may compete with all the strength of their manhood. We want to have free competition upwards; we decline to allow free competition to run downwards.'[107] The aim of Beveridge's plan for social insurance was quite simply 'to make want under any circumstances unnecessary'.[108] 'In the total outlay directed to maintaining full employment, priority is required for a minimum for all citizens of housing, health, education and nutrition, and a minimum of investment to raise the standard of life of future generations.'[109] It was definitely not, however, the responsibility of government to provide more than a minimum. Compulsory contributions to provide more than a minimum would, in Beveridge's view, be an attack on the individual's freedom to spend his money as he thinks best.[110] A national minimum both abolished want and preserved the individual's liberty to provide, or not to provide, benefits for himself and his family over and above this.

Galbraith was prepared to go further than Beveridge and establish a guaranteed minimum income for those not at work which would force employers to raise wages to this level.[111] Beveridge was, of course, concerned with a subsistence minimum, Galbraith with relative poverty rather than subsistence, but Galbraith's willingness to use such a powerful weapon to raise low pay is in line with Beveridge's view that the state should use all available powers to abolish want subject only to the preservation of essential liberties.

Beveridge's main weapon in the struggle to secure a national minimum was insurance. Insurance appealed to him for a variety of reasons. It seemed to allow both a guaranteed minimum income and scope for individual saving and freedom of choice and it epitomised the organic relationship between the state, the individual and the voluntary organisation which was Beveridge's ideal. Furthermore, social insurance raised no party political issues and this seemed to give his plan a strong chance of being implemented.

For Beveridge, however, the ultimately decisive argument for contributory insurance was that it was the only way to secure benefits as of right without a means test.[112] The avoidance of a means test was very important because such tests discourage voluntary insurance and saving. Thrift is important in itself and it is economically important if a larger proportion of the total savings of the community are going to have to come in the future from the modest savings of many citizens, rather than from the immodest savings of the few. To stimulate thrift, basic benefits must be granted without a means test.[113] A contributory scheme is also important to avoid the idea that the state is the dispenser of gifts for which no one needs to pay – a bottomless philanthropic purse.

While very aware of the limitations of voluntary insurance, Beveridge gave it an important place in his plan. It was essential in his view that the state scheme 'should leave room and encouragement for voluntary action by each individual to provide more than that minimum for himself and his family'.[114] Provision of benefit above subsistence level was an individual responsibility and it was the state's responsibility to ensure that its measures 'leave room and encouragement for such voluntary insurance'.[115] What Beveridge did, in fact, was to start from the centrality of a voluntary element and underpin it with a state scheme.

Beveridge's plea was for the state to assume a comprehensive approach to social welfare – hence the way he based his plan for social insurance on three assumptions – a National Health Service, a scheme of Family Allowances, and a policy of full employment. Removal of the economic barrier between patient and treatment was 'an essential negative step for bringing avoidable disease to an end', though positive steps to expand and develop preventive and curative facilities must follow.[116] He also made the obvious point that open access to medical care is a logical corollary of a state scheme for benefit during sickness. To let sickness continue for lack of treatment is an expense no government can afford. Family Allowances were a necessary element in any policy to secure a national minimum because the wages system on its own will not abolish poverty. A policy for full employment is required because simply to provide a subsistence income through insurance or assistance for those out of work is a totally inadequate provision for human happiness. The government should not feel that by making provision for income during unemployment it can avoid the prior responsibility of seeing that unemployment is reduced to a minimum.[117] Relief must be accompanied by treatment designed to cure the ills not simply to ease the pain.

The case which Beveridge argues for a wider state concern for welfare is not simply humanitarian. He also presses the argument that some welfare expenditure, for example on education, should be regarded as a communal investment, likely to bring a good return.[118] He argues the same investment case for Family Allowances. As regards unemployment benefit, he urges that provision on the most generous scale possible will help maintain purchasing power in depression, so mitigating its severity.[119]

Galbraith's attitude to the role of the state in welfare is pragmatic rather than ideological. He asserts the need for state responsibility, not as a matter of principle, but as a matter of necessity where other types of provision have failed. This is the burden of his argument for the New Socialism. He believes that an affluent society, by its very nature, increases the need for welfare intervention – for example, to care for the children whose mothers have returned to work so that they can buy the goods which industry must produce and sell if full employment is to be maintained, or to combat the lawlessness to which affluent societies seem prone,[120] or to provide medical treatment for the health hazards generated by affluence – obesity, cirrhosis, accidents due to increased consumption of alcohol, lung cancer, heart disease, nervous diseases, and so on.[121]

Public intervention and provision develop because the very changes which increase the need for a wide range of welfare services at the same time render their effective private provision less likely. The growth industries – the planning system – seize the ear of the state and become the prime beneficiaries of increased public spending. Public policy is geared to serving their needs – through higher education designed to produce the skills they require, through direct and indirect subsidies, public investment and markets for products, rather than ensuring the effective operation of health or housing services. The result is the contrast between the squalor of public services serving the needy but powerless, and the affluence of services assisting the needy but powerful.

Galbraith's central concern is with poverty rather than inequality. He sees no prospect of the elimination of poverty simply through economic growth but sees social welfare services as a potentially powerful weapon against poverty. In his view better schools, school meals, maintenance grants for needy children, free health care and grants for retraining all have a part to play. So, too, have a prices and incomes policy with redistributive aims, measures to combat racial discrimination and minimum wage legislation. His proposals are often imaginative – for example, his proposal in *The Affluent Society*, long before positive discrimination became part of the conventional wisdom, that 'to eliminate poverty efficiently, we must, indeed, invest more than proportionately in the children of the poor community'.[122] His stress on achieving social balance rather than redistribution is an attempt to take welfare policy out of politics, to confine it to ills which all right-minded people recognise and deplore.

The Social Democratic strand in reluctant collectivist thinking reflects both new and old perspectives. There is the acceptance of a mixed economy of welfare, private and public. Objection to private medicine, for example, is pragmatic not of principle. What is wrong is not the existence of private medicine as such but the ways its growth may distort the rational allocation of skilled people and specialist facilities.[123] The answer to the growth of the private sector is to improve the quality and quantity of public provision.

Another old emphasis in reluctant collectivism, revived in Social Democratic thinking, is the primacy given to an attack on poverty as the central function of the welfare state. The test of a just society, Owen has argued, is not the level of inequality which exists but how the poor fare. So a just society might be extremely unequal. The test by which welfare state policies are to be judged is narrowed to the question of whether they promote the interests of the worst off. Universalist policies often fail such a test.[124]

What is new is the stress on the need to decentralise and democratise the planning and control of public welfare and to reduce the role of central government in welfare provision. If the community is to be encouraged to take more responsibility for the standard of its health and social services, responsibility must be decentralised. An unelected centralist authority, Owen argues, is incapable of facing up to local problems and settling issues of priorities.[125]

The reluctant collectivists accept the desirability and necessity of state involvement in welfare provision on the grounds of the failure of other mechanisms of provision, the needs of society and the needs of individuals. They retain, however, a degree of anxiety about state monopoly and prefer a mixed economy of welfare with private and voluntary provision alongside public. They also remain more critical of the effectiveness and costs of state provisions than the Fabians.[126]

The overall aim of the reluctant collectivists is to purge capitalism of its inefficiencies and injustices so that it may survive. They believe in capitalism as potentially the most efficient form of economic organisation but they see it as doomed unless reformed and regulated. They believe that capitalism and planning are compatible, that government intervention is necessary to make capitalism morally acceptable and that such intervention is a practical proposition. The good things of capitalism can be preserved – most obviously its capacity for wealth creation – and its unacceptable face wiped clean.

In the early 1970s the reluctant collectivists and the Fabians seemed together to have reformed and saved capitalism. The mixed economy seemed very different from the economic system which had shocked Keynes and Beveridge into re-examining its foundations. It was clearly more successful and seemed more stable. Ten years later reluctant collectivists and Fabians are under attack, their achievements a fading memory and their ideas in disrepute – for the time being at least.

4

The Fabian socialists

There are many varieties of socialism. Crick, for example, identified five different schools[1] and Berki outlined four variations on the basic theme.[2] In spite of, or because of, this vagueness, socialism has a strong appeal to many people in many countries at all levels of economic development in all parts of the globe. In this, and the next chapter, we examine the two most important approaches to socialism and social welfare – Fabianism and Marxism.

The Fabian socialists occupy a substantial area of rather muddy middle ground between the reluctant collectivists and the Marxists. At the boundaries, the divisions between this group and their neighbours are sometimes blurred, and trespassing is quite frequent. The group contains a range of political and theoretical positions on socialism. For some it is a form of developed social democracy, to others it is only a few steps away from Marxist socialism. In spite of these differences, there are two unifying links in Fabianism: total commitment to the democratic process and unequivocal support for social welfare services.

Social values

Because of the importance they attach to the role of ideas and ideals in history, Fabians have a lot to say about the kind of social values which they consider essential to socialism and how these

69

differ from capitalist values. They stress three central values –
equality, freedom and fellowship – and two derivative values –
democratic participation which is the child of equality and
freedom and humanitarianism which is the offspring of equality
and fellowship. This is not an exhaustive list nor do all Fabians
describe the values in the same terms. Sometimes, too, there is
much more stress on one or two of these values than on others
but together these five make up the basic value-mix of British
democratic socialism.

The emphasis on equality comes from all wings of Fabianism –
the social democratic, the ethical and the semi-Marxist. Equality,
says Crosland, 'has been the strongest ethical inspiration of
virtually every socialist doctrine [and] still remains the most
characteristic feature of socialist thought today'.[3] For Tawney,
equality was also quite fundamental – 'the necessary corollary . . . of the Christian conception of man'.[4] Meacher insists
that gross inequality in capitalist societies is legitimated by a
series of 'myths' which must be exposed for what they are in
order to make possible the acceptance of equality – an essential
component of socialist ideology.[5]

The case for equality rests on four inter-related grounds –
social integration, economic efficiency, natural justice and
individual self-realisation. They are supported by a mixture of
pragmatic and ethical arguments and they have remained
remarkably unchanged over the seventy-year period which spans
the writings of Tawney and Townsend.

Tawney, Titmuss, Crosland and others saw a reduction of
inequality as a necessary, though not a sufficient, condition for
social integration and social harmony. Tawney, writing in a more
turbulent period, was deeply concerned about the problem of
social integration. In 1913 he spoke of his belief in equality as
'the one foundation of human subordination, of order, authority
and justice'.[6] Reduction of inequalities creates a greater feeling
of social belonging which, in turn, protects the social order
against violent upheavals. Even during the post-war years, when
British society was perhaps at its most orderly, Crosland sought
to explain the continuing existence of 'so many touchy, prickly,
indignant and frustrated citizens in politics and industry' by 'that
resentment against social inequality which is characteristic of
class antagonism'.[7] He explained that resentment in terms of
society's failure to assimilate new economic groups who, as a
result, found their social aspirations blocked. It was not merely a
question of personal frustration but of resentment felt by groups
of working-class people, which was made more serious because it

could threaten 'other exceedingly important values – democracy, social and industrial peace, tolerance and even personal free-dom'.[8] Titmuss, too, shared this view. 'History suggests', he wrote, 'that human nature is not strong enough to maintain itself in true community where great disparities of income and wealth preside.'[9]

The argument that inequality leads to general economic inefficiency is based on two main grounds. First, that massive inequalities lead to a misdirection of productive effort because the private market responds to demand rather than need. These can, at times, be the same but they can also be very different. Pronounced inequalities in a free market system can, therefore, lead to the production of cake for some before bread for all, of yachts and Rolls Royces before houses. Second, there is the argument that gross inequality creates inefficiency because it results in a waste of ability and talent. Crosland expresses one aspect of this when he says:

> If social mobility is low, as it must be in a stratified society, and people cannot easily move up from the lower or middle reaches to the top, then the ruling elite becomes hereditary and self-perpetuating; and whatever one may concede to inherited or family advantages, this must involve a waste of talent.[10]

The economic prosperity of a country depends, however, not only on the quality of the ruling élite but also on the quality of management and labour. Wastage of ability in any area of society is, therefore, to be deplored for economic reasons.

Gross inequalities offend against ideas of natural justice because they lead to a denial of natural rights when, for example, educational opportunities are distributed not according to ability but according to the accidents of birth and parental income. They also violate ideas of natural justice because they give certain groups immense power over others and because they endow a minority lavishly, not as a result of its contribution to the common good but because of birth or inheritance. Clearly, the basis of this objection is the assumption that all human beings have certain natural rights which should be respected by society.

The final argument for equality is a variant of the natural rights argument but it is presented separately because of the emphasis accorded to it in the writings of Tawney. Only in a more equal society, he argued, does the individual have the opportunity to realise his or her full potential. A society is civilised, Tawney insisted, in so far as it uses its material resources to provide for the dignity and refinement of the individual human beings who compose it. 'Violent contrasts of wealth and power and an undiscriminating devotion to institutions by which such contrasts are maintained and heightened do not promote the attainment of such ends but thwart it.'[11] Inequality thus diminishes people's basic humanity.

Though there is wide agreement on the basis of the case for greater economic and social equality, there is a great deal of disagreement and confusion among Fabians about the meaning of equality. Tawney, though arguing for reductions of wealth and income inequalities, was unwilling to be specific about what level of inequality was acceptable, and he was certainly against equality of incomes – for two main reasons. First, because he believed that: 'No one thinks it inequitable that when a reasonable provision has been made for all, exceptional responsibilities should be compensated by exceptional rewards as a recognition of the service performed and an inducement to perform it.'[12] Second, because he saw that the achievement and preservation of equality of incomes would require such massive government regulation that it could not be maintained in a free, democratic society.

Crosland's approach is similar to Tawney's in the sense that he, too, is against excessive stress on income inequality and he, too, brushes aside the question of how much equality is desirable. However, he differs from Tawney in two respects. He is more concerned with the effects of egalitarian measures on work incentives to the extent that he felt 'a definite limit exists to the degree of equality which is desirable'.[13] Second, and perhaps as a result, he is more concerned with the ways in which income inequalities arise than with the inequalities themselves. What is fundamentally unjust about the present pattern of income distribution, in his view, is the absence of an equal opportunity of attaining the top rewards. 'The essential thing', he writes,

> is that every citizen should have an equal chance – that is his basic democratic right; but provided the start is fair, let there be the maximum scope for individual self-advancement. There would then be nothing improper in either a high continuous status ladder (e.g. of income or consumption patterns) or even a distinct class stratification (e.g. a segregated education system), since opportunities for attaining the highest status or the topmost stratum would be genuinely equal.[14]

Crosland does not, surprisingly, perceive the crucial weakness in his argument that true equality of opportunity is simply not feasible in an unequal society either in the field of education or occupation. This is particularly important because of his views on wealth. Though he finds the existing distribution of wealth 'flagrantly unjust',[15] he does not condemn inequalities of wealth in principle. It is the origins of such inequalities which make them acceptable or unacceptable. In his view, wealth inequalities may be considered unjust on three grounds: if they stem from inherited property and not from work; if they reflect differences in opportunity rather than differences in ability; and if they are the product of unequally generous treatment by the tax system.[16]

Meacher, writing from a left-wing position, also feels that it is not practical politics to specify in advance the degree of income inequalities which would be acceptable in a socialist society, apart from stating that it will be lower than it is in contemporary Britain. Some types and degrees of inequality are acceptable in a socialist society. The important thing is that 'the institutions of society ought to work towards reducing them [inequalities of income] provided that the basic liberties of each individual are not improperly infringed'.[17] Both Townsend and Walker, however, are prepared to be more specific in this area: they both argue for a minimum and a maximum wage and Townsend couples this with the suggestion that maximum gross earnings should not be more than four times the average male wage.[18]

Fabian socialists differ, as we said earlier, in the relative priority they give to different values. Crosland saw equality as 'the strongest ethical inspiration of virtually every socialist doctrine'.[19] Roy Jenkins, in his Fabian days, agreed.[20] Frank Field, however, has argued more recently that freedom, which we now come on to discuss, is the central socialist value and greater equality is no more than a means to that end – though a vital means.[21]

Three elements in particular distinguish the Fabian socialist conception of freedom from that of the anti-collectivists. First, a belief in freedom means, as a necessary corollary, a concern for equality. Freedom depends on a reduction of inequality because if there are major inequalities of resources or of economic power, some men are in bondage to others. The fundamental idea of liberty, says Tawney, is power to control the conditions of one's own life – and this means economic equality.[22]

Second, the idea of freedom is as relevant to the work situation as it is in the political sphere. Economic freedom, according to Crosland, means that workers should have a voice in the conditions of their work, that they should be recognised as possessing certain rights in relation to it, and that employers should not be able to exercise arbitrary power of regulation or dismissal over them.[23] Some go even further to argue for workers' control rather than workers' participation in industry, as we shall see in a later section of the chapter.

Third, freedom is the product of government action rather than government inaction. This is so because freedom is defined to mean not simply freedom from but freedom for as well. 'Home-made socialism', writes Field, when discussing measures to reduce inequality and abolish poverty, 'is essentially about extending freedom, not of the few but of the many.'[24] He and all other Fabians will agree with Tawney's assessment in 1949 that: 'The increase in the freedom of ordinary men and women during the last two generations has taken place, not in spite of the action of governments, but because of it. . . . The mother of liberty has, in fact, been law.'[25]

Among Fabian socialists there is substantial agreement with Beer's conclusion that though the socialist system of values includes equality and liberty, 'one gets at the heart of its ethical message with the concept of fellowship'.[26] By fellowship or fraternity, the socialist means cooperation rather than competition, an emphasis on duties rather than rights, on the good of the community rather than on the wants of the individual, on altruism rather than on selfishness. From all wings of Fabianism, fellowship emerges as a dominant value.

The basis of Tawney's critique of the acquisitive society is the way in which it invites and encourages men and women to use the power and skills with which they have been endowed solely for their own profit rather than for the good of their fellow human beings as well. It is not simply a matter of individual predisposition, but of a capitalist system which creates and fosters such attitudes and behaviour, which treats people 'not as human personalities, but as tools, not as ends, but as means'.[27] A new social order – a socialist society – would provide the institutional framework for a new set of right relationships among its citizens. In such a society people will regard themselves 'not primarily as the owners of rights but as trustees for the discharge of functions and the instruments of a social purpose'.[28] People will come to view the rights they possess in relation to the duties they must perform for the sake of the good of all in society.

Titmuss's emphasis on altruism and giving to strangers is the essence of a true social service and of a socialist society. If Tawney's emphasis is on the institutional arrangements, Titmuss's is on the personal willingness of individuals to behave altruistically to others by supporting a universal range of social services. This was important for otherwise society would be dominated by self-interest and conflict. 'There is nothing permanent', he writes, 'about the expressing of reciprocity. If the bonds of community giving are broken, the result is not a state of value neutralism. The vacuum is likely to be filled by hostility and social conflict.'[29]

More recently, Meacher puts fellowship at the top of the socialist value hierarchy, even though the words he uses to describe it are different. While capitalism runs, he argues, on the values of élitism, materialism and competitiveness, socialism must rely on 'the values of sharing, altruism, and cooperation'.[30] He is aware, however, of the immense difficulties involved in the transformation of a capitalist ethic into a socialist ethic and he calls for educational and other measures to help bring it about.

As mentioned earlier, Fabians have argued that political freedom needs to be complemented with economic freedom in order to have real meaning for all members of society. Their emphasis on democratic participation is an extension of this belief that political democracy is only one element in a truly democratic society. It follows from this that democratic participation in all aspects of life – not only in politics and at the work place – is, in Durbin's words, 'an inherent part of socialism'.[31] In a later section, we shall see how the notion of democratic participation is applied to the social services.

Finally, Fabian socialists have stressed the value of humanitarianism – a deep concern that people should be able to enjoy certain minimum standards of life and that social distress should be swept away. Thus, they give an exceptionally high priority to traditional social welfare goals and to the devotion of an increased proportion of the national income to such goals. Crosland sees this as practical and non-doctrinal and considers it 'much the most powerful inspiration from the earliest days of the Labour Party'.[32] He emphasises that it is humanitarianism not egalitarianism which has been the main driving force behind the efforts of the Labour movement to create a welfare state. Titmuss adds another dimension to humanitarianism by his insistence that it means giving priority to the welfare of deprived minorities. It means, therefore, that we should spend proportionately more on the educationally deprived than on the educationally normal, press forward with the rehousing of the poor more rapidly than with the housing of the better off, and devote proportionately more medical services to the needs of the chronic sick than to those of the average sick.[33]

Society and the state

Apart from occasional lapses, Fabian socialists see society as made up of classes and groups whose interests are in conflict. They differ from Marxists in that they do not consider class conflict as paramount and all other types of conflict as derivative and secondary. According to the Fabian view, only a close analysis of a particular situation can decide which form of conflict is paramount. Nevertheless, there are substantial differences among Fabians in the importance they attribute to class conflict, to the power of the capitalist class and to the nature of the state. The views of Tawney, Crosland and Meacher are discussed here because they represent different positions within Fabianism – ethical socialism, social democracy and semi-Marxist socialism. The choice of authors is dictated also by the reluctance among Fabian socialists to theorise. Kincaid's comment on Titmuss – 'the reader cannot expect to find . . . any overall consistency of theoretical or political position'[34] – applies to many other Fabians.

Tawney claimed that the private ownership of the means of production and distribution had two inevitable consequences for the structure of society. First, it leads to 'the creation of a class of pensioners upon industry, who levy toll upon its product, but contribute nothing to its increase and who are not merely tolerated, but applauded and admired and protected with assiduous care, as though the secret of prosperity resided in them'. Second, it results in 'the degradation of those who labour, but who do not by their labour command large rewards; that is of the great majority of mankind'.[35] This division of society into classes inevitably leads to class conflict even though the form it takes varies a great deal. Tawney's discussion of class conflict identifies two important features: first, that such conflict is perpetual 'though not always obtrusive, [it] is active below the surface',[36] and second, that it is natural, and is 'not caused by a misunderstanding of identity of interests but by a better understanding of diversity of interests'.[37] In such a society, it is idle for governments to talk about 'the national interest' and to appeal to workers to make sacrifices for it. The fact is, Tawney insisted, that

> there is not one society but two which dwell together in uneasy juxtaposition, like Sinbad and the Old Man of the Sea, but which in spirit, in ideals, and in economic interest, are worlds

asunder. There is the society of those who live by labour, whatever their craft or profession, and the society of those who live on it.[38]

In spite of the interlocking of élites and the powerful position of the capitalist class, which he identified,[39] Tawney rejected the Marxist idea that the state was simply the executive committee of the capitalist class. 'The state', he wrote, 'is an important instrument; hence the struggle to control it. But it is an instrument and nothing more. Fools will use it, when they can, for foolish ends, criminals for criminal ends. Sensible and decent men will use it for ends which are sensible and decent.'[40] There is a genuine break here with Marxist thinking on the nature of the state – discussed in the following chapter – but part of this difference of opinion is also due to different definitions of the state. Tawney implies that the state is equivalent to the government, the civil service and the judiciary, whereas for Marxists the state is far more encompassing. The wider the view taken of the state, the more difficult it becomes for governments to control it.

It followed from Tawney's position that a Labour government could use the state machinery to introduce radical changes. Inevitably, the capitalist class would attempt to block such changes but a determined government would secure its aims. It would not be an easy or a civilised process but, with public opinion behind a radical programme, the government could probably impose its will on the capitalist class.

His deep religious beliefs and his strong commitment to democracy led Tawney away from the use of violence to achieve political ends, however desirable such ends might seem. He was sure that the British public would not countenance the use of violence and he was equally certain that violence would contaminate socialism – ends and means could not be divorced. The only justification for the use of force by a government was to defeat an attempt at its own overthrow. In all other circumstances, democratic means were the only acceptable method for the achievement of socialism. And when socialism is achieved, democracy will flourish more healthily than under capitalism. Terrill sums up the centrality of the democratic road to socialism for Tawney when he writes that he felt that 'not only no other path can bring socialism, but that the so-called path is actually part of the destination'.[41]

Crosland's analysis of the capitalist system in the 1950s was very different from Tawney's in the 1920s. Unlike Tawney, who thought capitalism was breaking down, Crosland felt that capitalism had been transformed into a stable economic and political system and he even gave it a new name – statism. As he put it, 'by 1951 Britain had, in all the essentials, ceased to be a capitalist country' and 'statism represents a major social revolution. . . . With its arrival, the most characteristic features of capitalism have all disappeared'.[42]

Nevertheless, classes still existed in British society and he accepted as inevitable the divergence of class interests and the conflict, actual or potential, between the two sides of industry. However, the picture he painted of class conflict was less clear cut than that described by Tawney. He talked of 'a disturbing amount of . . . social antagonism and class resentment, visible both in politics and industry',[43] though by the 1970s he was prepared to accept that the scope and intensity of class conflict was greater than he had originally thought. 'Class relations in industry', he wrote in 1974, 'are characterised by a mutual distrust amounting often to open warfare.'[44]

Crosland's analysis of the class structure of British society led him naturally to the rejection of the Marxist view of the state. The capitalist class, he argued, could no longer dictate policies to governments, as it did in the 1930s – rather the reverse was the case in the 1950s. There were three reasons for this transformation of the balance of power in British political life: first, the nationalisation measures and other achievements of the Labour government of 1945-51 which resulted in more economic power being transferred from private hands to the government; second, the growth of trade union power which resulted from full employment; and third, the change in attitudes among the capitalist class which came about as a result of the managerial revolution – the shift of power from owners to managers. Private industry had become more civilised and humanised.[45] Crosland saw this transformation in political power as permanent and irreversible. His faith in government's ability to impose its policies on a reluctant capitalist class remained undaunted even after the Labour government had had to change or abandon some of its policies in the 1960s in the face of opposition from private enterprise. He attributed that setback to lack of will on the government's part, rather than to the strength of the forces opposing it.[46] He continued to regard the parliamentary road to socialism as quite feasible with fewer obstacles than Tawney envisaged. Like Tawney, of course, he saw democracy and socialism not only as compatible but as inseparable and as mutually enriching.

The differences between Tawney and Crosland may have been due partly to the fact that they lived and wrote during very different times: Tawney, at times of high unemployment, low wages and massive poverty; Crosland during the full employment period of the 1950s and 1960s. It is noticeable, however, that Crosland's writings during the 1970s became less optimistic about a socialist future. By the late 1970s, many of Crosland's claims – permanent full employment, strong trade unionism, the abolition of poverty – had been proved, if not totally wrong, to be no more than half-truths.

Unlike Crosland, who maintained that the capitalist class had weakened during the post-war period, Meacher holds that its power has increased. The growth of near monopolies and of multi-national companies has meant that economic power has become more concentrated and hence more influential in dealings with governments. The implication of this, claims Meacher, is that government has to take account of the interests of these powerful big businesses. Collapse of a large national industry has implications for employment, wages, government tax revenues, and so on. In this way, 'the "national interest" becomes automatically identified with the health and prosperity of the dominant companies. . .'.[47] The power of the financial sector of the capitalist class has also grown with equally serious implications for government policies. The City of London, for example, has increasingly forced governments to deal with successive economic crises in such a way that 'the City's priorities have predominated, gradually at first, but more strongly and overtly later'.[48] The composition and the internal workings of the top echelons of the civil service also lend support to the socio-economic system. Senior civil servants exercise substantial influence over ministers and government policies. 'The slant of this power, while normally not conspiratorial or anti-reformist, is certainly ideologically towards the maintenance, albeit with improved operation, of the existing socio-economic system.'[49]

These three pivots of the British power structure, Meacher argues, are not three separate social groups. They are united by family background and education; they are linked by cross-membership; and they have common economic interests. The result is not three separate élites but one ruling class with massive economic and political power. In such circumstances, the state is not an impartial arbiter among competing interests. Rather it 'is primarily and inevitably the guardian and protector of the economic interests that predominate in it. Its real function is to ensure their continued dominance, not to over-ride them.'[50]

Meacher's approach is similar to Tawney's in one respect – his belief in the existence of a capitalist class with massive economic and political power – but different in another – the view that the power of this class is so overwhelming that governments, to a greater or lesser extent, become its willing or unwilling protector. This view of the state is similar to the Marxist 'relative autonomy' thesis discussed in the next chapter. Yet Meacher sees the road to socialism as peaceful and democratic in spite of all the difficulties and problems involved. In brief, the belief in democracy as the only road towards, and as the essence of socialism, is deeply ingrained in Fabian thinking of all political shades.

In spite of their differing analyses of capitalism, Fabian socialists show a high level of agreement in the criticism they make of the free market system. Their charges can be grouped under five headings: The first is that it is unethical and this charge represents the heart of Tawney's attack on acquisitive societies. It is that

> the motive which gives colour and quality to their public institutions, to their policy and political thought, is not the attempt to secure the fulfilment of tasks undertaken for the public service but to increase the opportunities open to individuals of attaining the objects which they conceive to be advantageous to themselves.[51]

It is a system which excludes consideration of collective goals because the only acceptable collective goal is that individuals should be free to pursue their own interests. In such a society there can be no clear social purpose. The result is, at best, an uneven pattern of public services, at worst, avoidable ills and public squalor.

The second charge is that the market system is fundamentally unjust. It distributes its rewards on no clear principles and this lack of principle is inevitable in a society where each individual has a prescriptive moral right to what he can extract from his fellow citizens without contravening the law.[52] It is, therefore, natural that in such a society gross injustices will always exist and will be generally accepted.

Third, the market system is undemocratic. Decisions important to many individuals are taken either in the gilded privacy of the corridors of power to which the majority have no access, or are not taken at all, but left to the capricious whim of market forces. It is on the first count that Titmuss indicts the private insurance companies because they constitute a major shift in economic power in our society. It is a power, a potential power, to affect many important aspects of our economic life and our social values. . . . It is power concentrated in relatively few hands, working at the apex of a handful of giant bureaucracies, technically supported by a group of professional experts, and accountable, in practice, to virtually no one.[53]

The fourth charge is that the free market is inefficient unless regulated by government. If left to itself, private enterprise leads to ecological devastation, to the social blight of some regions and urban areas, to periodic, slumps, to excessive production of fundamentally useless products and inadequate production or supply of socially necessary goods and services – all of which have detrimental effects on both economic development and the quality of life. The fifth and final charge made against the free market system is that the pattern of distribution of the national product to which it leads is, as Titmuss put it, 'out of sympathy with the contemporary distribution of social need arising from the dependencies of childhood, widowhood, sickness and old age'.[54]

The role of government

Given their social values and their criticisms of capitalist society, how do Fabian socialists hope to see their ideal society realised? The answer is through purposeful government action. The task of government is to modify the injustices of the private market system. The socialists' concern for welfare and equality lead to a particular view of collective responsibility. This, says Crosland, 'represents the first major difference between a socialist and a conservative'.[55] As we shall be discussing the social services in the next section, we will concentrate here on economic policy. Government planning, it is believed, can transform capitalism into socialism without endangering individual freedom as the anti-collectivists maintain. In opposition to the belief that planning is the road to serfdom, Fabians feel that 'it is as possible to plan for freedom as for tyranny'.[56] Like the Marxists, Fabians reject the notion that minimum government intervention is essential to the maintenance of freedom. Rather, they believe, the opposite, that government action is necessary to modify the market concentration of power and to extend power to the wider public. In Tawney's words, if freedom implies, as presumably it does, the possession by individuals of a genuine, if partial, power of self-determination, then, so far from having been attenuated by measures conducive to the more general enjoyment of physical and mental vitality, it has gained in substance and reality as a result of them.[57]

What is important is that the democratic parliamentary process controls planning so that the power of the government and its officials remains always answerable to the public.

What type of government economic measures are necessary then to transform capitalist society? The nationalisation of the means of production and distribution has always been a central plank of the Fabian programme. All the Fabians of the 1930s saw this as indispensable, though there are different views about the form nationalisation could take and it was seen as only one of several ways in which private enterprise could be 'socialised'. Tawney referred to six different ways in which 'the dead hand of private ownership' could be removed,[58] and deplored the fact that so much attention was focussed on nationalisation only. Workers' cooperatives, consumers' associations, government regulation, control and ownership of private enterprise were all suggested as alternatives to nationalisation. Basically, Tawney's point was that all forms of 'socialisation' measures were means to an end – the end being 'to release those who do constructive work from the control of those whose sole interest is pecuniary gain, in order that they may be free to apply their energies to the true purpose of industry, which is the provision of services not the provision of dividends'.[59] The decision as to which of these different forms of socialisation was appropriate should be decided on pragmatic grounds depending on the circumstances of each industry.

The debate on the nationalisation issue has continued over the years so that Fabians today are divided between 'revisionists' and 'fundamentalists'. The fundamentalists believe that the widespread extension of public ownership is necessary for the achievement of socialism, while the revisionists feel that welfare capitalism can be tamed and harnessed to socialist aims with only limited extension of public ownership. Crosland argued against extensive nationalisation and felt that even where nationalisation was necessary, it should be selective, taking over individual firms while leaving others in private hands, or setting up new government-owned plants to compete with existing private firms.[60] For the revisionists, the mixed economy becomes the end of the road rather than simply a staging post. It is a far cry from Tawney's eloquent indictments of the very nature of capitalism and from Meacher's economic programme that deals with imports and exports, production targets, planning enterprise boards, and so on – what has come to be known as the alternative economic strategy.[61]

Discussion of the extension of public ownership has always been accompanied by a debate on the extension of public participation in decision-making. If actively pursued, it was felt in the 1930s, it would have economic, social and political benefits. It would help to spread responsibility, reduce power concentration and increase productivity. While participation was possible within limits in private industry, only in 'socialised' industries was it possible for it to reach its full potential. These aspirations of the Fabians of the 1930s did not materialise in the nationalised industries created by the Labour Government of 1945-51. It was left to Crosland to point out that nationalisation 'is no panacea for bad relations' in industry[62] and to argue that the value of workers' participation had been exaggerated. Nevertheless, during the late 1970s, with the general realisation that nationalisation does not reduce concentration of economic power, participation has come to be seen again as one of the central elements of socialism. Indeed, there are those few among Fabian socialists who believe that real participation is only possible if practised at the local grass roots level. Luard is an example of this minority view. 'The first requirement' for a new socialist beginning, he writes,

> is to develop the concept of socialism at the *grass roots*: of social ownership and socialist organisation on a small scale in the local unit; in the municipality rather than the state, the enterprise, or even the workshop, rather than the national industry; in the school, the housing association, the community centre, rather than in the society as a whole.[63]

In brief, the issue of participation has proved troublesome and elusive but it is still at the centre of Fabian economic strategy for a socialist society – just as it is among Marxists, as we shall see in the next chapter.

Gross inequalities of income and wealth have been condemned by Fabians of all political shades, as pointed out earlier in this chapter. It comes as no surprise, therefore, that all Fabians have argued over the years for taxation policies that reduce such inequalities and make the inheritance of large fortunes imposs-ible. What divides Fabians is the extent to which wealth and profits should be taxed. Again, the division between 'revisionists' and 'fundamentalists' comes to the surface. According to Crosland,

> The problem facing British socialists is therefore so to use our democratic institutions as to ensure that profit in the private sector is used primarily for re-investment, and not . . . for distribution to private shareholders. . . . Naturally share-holders are entitled to an income commensurate with the risks entailed in investment.[64]

He adopts similarly mild policies towards the taxation of wealth, particularly wealth that has not been inherited. This is a different approach from that of Townsend, for example, who argues that the 'wealth of the rich must be substantially reduced . . . and a statutory definition of maximum permissible wealth in relation to the minimum agreed'. He also makes similar recommendations in relation to top salaries or wages.[65] Experience over the last forty years shows that neither the nationalisation nor the taxation measures adopted so far have had much impact on the extent of wealth inequalities apart from some redistribution from the extremely rich to the very rich.

Fabian socialists will claim that their distinctive contribution to the welfare of the British public has been their championship of the social services. Before we go on to examine their general position on social policy, it is important to refer to the increasing realisation among Fabians that economic policies have direct and indirect effects on social policy and vice-versa. To quote Townsend again: 'the management of an economy is inseparable from its social effects. It is impossible to have an economic policy . . . which is not also a social policy.'[66] It is out of this realisation that suggestions have been made by several Fabians for the formulation of an alternative social policy to partner the alternative economic policy – both of which will contest the market-centred economic policies and the residual social policies of the anti-collectivists.

The welfare state

How do Fabian socialists explain the development of the welfare state? How do they view the functions and nature of the social services? How do social services as currently organised differ from how Fabians see socialist social services? These are the three main questions to be discussed in this section.

The development of the welfare state has not so far been adequately conceptualised by Fabian socialists. What one finds in their writings are passing comments which are occasionally contradictory and do not add up to a theoretical position. Tawney's explanation was both brief and simple. In agricultural societies there is neither the wealth nor the collective perception of the need for social services. It is industrialisation which creates the right conditions for the emergence of social services. On one hand, it concentrates, increases and highlights social problems – crime, illiteracy, poverty and disease, for example – through rapid and unplanned urbanisation. On the other hand, it creates the wealth that is necessary to finance collective responses to such problems. When political awareness and social scientific knowledge develop, then the pressure for government action increases. Tawney sums it up as follows: 'The causes of the movement are not obscure. It is the natural consequence of the simultaneous development of an industrial civilisation and of political democracy.'[67] One can read as much or as little into this as one likes, but what is clear is that Tawney did not give much thought to the precise relationships between the various factors which he mentions. In another passage he likens the social services to 'rudimentary communism' and concludes that it all happened accidentally. 'The rise of this rudimentary communism has taken place without design and almost unconsciously, as a method of coping with grave practical evils.'[68]

Marshall's thesis that the growth of legal and political rights both preceded and created the right conditions for the growth of social rights as an aspect of evolving citizenship in industrial societies is another approach that belongs to the Fabian school. It is similar to Tawney's in one respect – it takes a long view of social policy development without too much concern about detailed evidence – but it is different in another. It sees social services as an outgrowth of democracy rather than as a response to pressures for socialism or a step in that direction.[69] Crosland, too, subscribes to the citizenship view in his discussion of the movement for comprehensive education. 'Over the past 300 years', he wrote, 'these rights [of citizenship] have been extended first to personal liberty then to political democracy, and later to social welfare. Now they must be further extended to educational equality.'[70] What is missing from this approach, however, is an attempt to discuss the specific forces fuelling the movement for social services.

It is to Titmuss that one turns to fill this gap. But what one finds is a number of brief discussions of specific cases of policy development but the discussions take place in a theoretical vacuum. The result is that different inferences can be drawn depending on the particular case examined. Usually he adopts a social class and pressure group conflict model of society to explain the development of social policy. There are, however, exceptions; for example, his statement that

> All collectively provided services are deliberately designed to meet certain socially recognised 'needs'; they are manifestations, first, of society's will to survive as an organic whole and, secondly, of the expressed wish of all the people to assist the survival of some people.[71]

Like Tawney, Titmuss sees the growth of the social services as the response to forces associated with the process of industrialisation but, like Tawney, he does not explain the precise nature of the forces or how they exert pressure. The fact that the growth of social services has taken place after countries have become industrialised is not in dispute. Evidence from comparative study attests to that. What is at issue is the reasons, the precise and specific ways in which industrialisation leads to the growth of social services.

Titmuss provides three answers, largely incompatible, in different parts of his writings. First, he sees social services as a bribe that the capitalist class is prepared to offer to the working class in return for social and political compliance.

> The aims and content of social policy both in peace and war are thus determined – at least to a substantial extent – by how far the cooperation of the masses is essential to the successful prosecution of war. If this cooperation is thought to be essential, then inequalities must be reduced, and the pyramid of social stratification must be flattened.[72]

He joins forces here with such right-wing politicians as Bismarck and with some Marxists who see social policy as the ransom volunteered by the capitalist state to undermine radical protest.

Second, he sees social policy development in exactly the opposite light – as part of the enlightened effort of the whole of society to alleviate distress so as to bring about a better, more united society. This comes out in the quotation given earlier describing social policy as the product of society's will to survive as an organic whole, as well as in his view that in the development of social services after the Second World War, 'the fundamental and dominating historical processes . . . were connected with the demand for one society'.[73]

Third, he sees the development of social services as the result of a complex web of interacting and interlocking forces. Thus he explains the growth of medical services as follows:

> Though the demand for social justice has been one of the major forces . . . other forces have played an equal – and sometimes more important – role. One . . . is the advancement of scientific knowledge. Another is represented by the movement from fatalism to awareness in popular attitudes towards health and disease. Yet another is the recurrent business of liberal thought to release the individual (whether in this context, doctor or patient) from unalterable dependence on any particular social group.[74]

Similarly, the growth of social security is attributed to several factors though this time they are mainly political rather than scientific and demographic.

> Fear of social revolution, the need for a law abiding labour force, the struggle for power between political parties and pressure groups, a demand to remove some of the social costs of change – for example, industrial accidents – from the back of the worker, and the social conscience of the rich – all played a part.[75]

Though one can find evidence to present Titmuss as a man of all seasons he was happier when he saw the development of social policy as the response of a complex network of factors produced by a particular situation. In this approach he represents the overall Fabian view of the development of the welfare state as a logical response to practical problems, as the product of the impact of industrialisation, urbanisation, technological change and democracy, and as the outcome of conflicting group interests as well as of general societal interests. This historical pragmatism was Titmuss's strength and his weakness.

How do Fabian socialists view the functions and nature of the social services? Generally, speaking, Fabian writers have given more thought to the functions of social policy than to its development though they do not always distinguish between its aims and its consequences. Nor is it always clear whether their references to aims and consequences refer to those actually existing or to the ideal, socialist ones.

Tawney referred to five overlapping aims of the social services but they can be better presented under three headings: the supply of basic necessities for all; the supplementation of a person's income from work with services according to need; and the encouragement of economic growth through improvement in human capital and through stabilising demand in the private market.[76] Crosland identified four similar functions of social expenditure: 'to relieve social distress and hardship and correct social need; to correct individual malfunctioning through social work intervention; to increase efficiency and reduce waste; and to improve social mixing and facilitate social mobility'.[77] Marshall argues along similar lines. Of the three types of aims which social policy can have – the elimination of poverty, the maximisation of welfare and the pursuit of equality – it is the second, he felt, that 'expresses the philosophy of the welfare state'.[78]

Titmuss referred at greater length to a multitude of functions which Wilding has grouped under six headings.[79] First, social services distribute and redistribute resources in a variety of ways and between a variety of groups. There is vertical and horizontal redistribution of income between socio-economic groups across the generations and between various status groups. Redistribution is thus an inevitable and proper function of social policy. Second, services act both as a positive force for social integration and as a negative force for social control. Titmuss, in his idealist moments, saw social policy as promoting the creation of a better and more harmonious society, one that approximated to a socialist society. At other times he recognised, as we pointed out earlier, that social reform was largely a kind of social tranquilliser. Third, social policy aimed at compensating individuals for the 'diswelfare' – the social injuries – they suffered as a result of economic changes in capitalist society. Titmuss also extended the notion of 'diswelfares' to cover injuries for which the industrial system was not responsible but which, nevertheless, were not the individual's own responsibility, for example, mental or physical handicap. Fourth, irrespective of their wide societal consequences, social services function to promote individual welfare. Without social services, social distress would be more widespread in society. Fifth, social services are a form of economic investment for both the individual and the nation. Sixth, social services provide channels for the social and biological need of individuals to help their fellow citizens.

Titmuss saw human beings not as selfish by nature but rather as shaped by their social environment. 'If it is accepted', he concluded, 'that man has a social and biological need to help, then to deny him opportunities to express this need is to deny him the freedom to enter into gift relationships.' [80] Social services, in brief, help to promote altruism in society.

Not only is there no distinction between aims and consequences in this discussion but very little evidence is produced to substantiate the claims which are made. Moreover, there is hardly any discussion of the possible conflict between these various aims or functions. Indeed, several of the claims by their very nature can neither be proved nor disproved, while for others evidence is sparse, conflicting and inconclusive.[81]

To explore the Fabians' views on the nature of social services it is helpful to explore their stance in the universality-selectivity debate. This raises fundamental questions about the very nature of the role of the state in welfare. If the anti-collectivists have sided with selectivity, the Fabians have been on the side of universal social service provision. It is, perhaps, easier to present the Fabian position in this debate by presenting their reasons for disliking selectivity based on means tests. First, means tests can deter people from applying for services because of the inevitable complexity which results or because of public feelings about the stigmatising effects of tests. If means tests are intended to channel resources to those most in need, they fail to do this. Second, means tests can be used and are used to restrict demand rather than to meet need – a policy which is contrary to the very essence of a social service. Third, means tests create a climate of opinion which sees the users of the services as a burden on society and this gradually leads to the neglect of the services. Separate social services for the poor 'tend to become poor standard systems', claimed Titmuss.[82] The historical evidence about means-testing provides ample evidence for these criticisms.

The introduction of universal services by the Labour government in the immediate post-war years had the full backing of the Fabians. Titmuss argued that this was a necessary development in order to promote social integration, to break down 'distinctions and discriminative tests between first and second class citizens' and to provide equal opportunity of access to all. He was aware that equal access was different from equal outcome and understood that: 'Other and more precise instruments of social policy are required in addition to achieve equality of outcome irrespective of race, religion or class.'[83] But he was unwilling to accept individual means tests as a method of channelling more resources to the needy for the reasons given earlier. Instead, he argued for selective services based on either territorial criteria or client group criteria and operating within a framework of universal social services.

> The challenge that faces us is not the choice between universalist and selective services. The real challenge resides in the question: what particular infrastructure of universalist services is needed in order to provide a framework of values and opportunity bases within and around which can be developed acceptable selective services provided, as social rights, on criteria of the *needs* of specific categories, groups and territorial areas and not dependent on individual tests of means?[84]

Crosland was more accommodating, in principle, to the idea of means tests though his approach led in practice to a similar position to that of Titmuss. He argued strongly in favour of universal availability of services but he was not necessarily in favour of universal free availability. He emphasised the difference between a test of means, which determines the right to use a service, and one which simply determines the question of payment. In his view, an income test to determine whether access to the service should or should not be free was quite acceptable provided that two conditions were fulfilled. 'First, the benefit or service must not be so essential and so large in relation to the recipient's means that he may reasonably consider he has a social right to it, so that both his real income and self-esteem would be severely affected by a test of means.' This clearly rules out income tests for social security benefits and for most of education and health services. 'Secondly, the income-line should be as high as possible so that free services are not confined to the very poorest with all the stigmatising effects that this implies.'[85] The net result of these conditions is that free and universal social services will remain the dominant form of social provision but they will be supplemented at the margin by services based on generous income tests. Crosland's formula does not, of course, tackle the particular problems of the most deprived groups and areas which Titmuss attempts to solve.

Related to the universality-selectivity debate is the issue of the proper balance between public and private provision in the social services. Fabian socialists are agreed on the undesirable effects of private provision in education, health and social security. Such services increase inequality; they undermine altruism and social solidarity; they weaken public services; they concentrate power in private hands; and they are often parasitic on the public purse in direct and indirect ways. Fabians are agreed that the scope of private provision should be reduced but they disagree as to how best this can be done. There are those who would prohibit or abolish private provision in education and health by law,[86] but not social security. On the other hand, there are those who would prefer not to legislate but to make private provision unattractive by improving government services.[87] Lastly, there are those who would not legislate against private provision but who would financially and administratively make life very difficult for private social services.[88] Each position involves agonising choices between safeguarding the freedom of the few individuals who can afford to pay, and protecting the interests of the majority who cannot. Many of those who are against making private education or private medicine illegal are not necessarily less committed to the ideal of an egalitarian society – they are simply more cautious over the ethical and practical considerations involved. It must be conceded, however, that it is most unlikely for purely financial reasons that the standard of public services can ever be raised to that of private services. Similarly, it is difficult to imagine that those who so wish will not find ways round any administrative and fiscal impediments that a government may erect against private social services.

Fabian socialists have long been identified as the champions of the welfare state against the privatisation policies of the right and the denigrating commentary on the limitations of public welfare services from the Marxists. As far as the latter is concerned, Tawney's outburst fifty years ago will strike a chord of approval among Fabians today. 'To deprecate the social services as "mere palliatives"', he wrote, 'is a piece of clap-trap, which plays into the hands of the interests bent on saving the pockets of the rich at the expense of the children and the unemployed.'[89] While supporting the aims and purposes of the welfare state, socialists have remained aware of its limitations and dangers. They have voiced four general fears – that it is concerned with injustice and treatment rather than with justice and prevention; that it is too often limited to seeking equality of opportunity rather than pursuing equality of outcome; that it is concerned with poverty not with inequality; and that its administrative structures have been patronising and authoritarian rather than democratic and participative. We look at these fears in turn.

In the very early days of state welfare provision, Tawney pointed out the danger implicit in the social reformers' preoccupation with the exceptional misfortunes of life at the expense of an extension of the opportunity for the majority to live a life of security and independence.[90] Indeed, all the Fabian socialists of the 1930s were aware of the fact that social services would not, by themselves, provide a socially just society. They could only do that if they operated within an economic system based on the socialisation of the means of production and distribution. The understandable euphoria surrounding the extension of the social services at the end of the Second World War concealed for a time the truth of this important warning – but not for long. In 1968, Titmuss reminded his audience of the narrow perspective which was being used to gauge the success of the welfare state. 'Thought, research and action have been focussed too heavily on the poor; poverty engineering has thus been abstracted from society. Social policy has been seen as an *ad hoc* appendage to economic growth, the provision of benefits, not the formulation of rights.'[91] By the 1980s, there was even greater understanding of the limitations of social policy in a hostile economic environment and there have been demands that the working out of an effective radical social policy be given equal priority with the development of new economic strategy. Policies based simply on the notion of equality of opportunity, claim the Fabians, are not the answer to inequality. In the first place, equality of opportunity is not attainable in a society where people's circumstances are so unequal from the moment of birth. In the second place, socialists should be aspiring to equality of outcome rather than simply the opportunity for an equal race.

While the abolition of poverty is crucial to socialists they obviously do not see it as being a satisfactory ultimate objective. Poverty and inequality are seen as aspects of the same problem and the elimination of the former is seen as needing to be accompanied by the substantial reduction of the latter. It is now generally agreed, among Fabians, that whatever else it has achieved, the advent of the 'welfare state' in Britain after the Second World War has not led to any significant vertical redistribution of wealth or income.[92]

The 1970s saw an increasing concern among Fabians about the nature of social service bureaucracies. Three related charges have been laid against them: that they are too centralised and hierarchical; that they confer too much power on the pro-fessionals and the administrators; and that they allow very little, if any, say to the users of the service. Crosland argued that local authorities should give the council tenant a security, an independence, and a freedom to do what he likes in his house, which is comparable to that of the owner occupier. A programme for greater tenants' democracy should, therefore, form a central and probably the most novel part of a Labour housing programme.[93]

Similar calls have been made in relation to the other social services.

Until recently there was a marked tendency among Fabians to attribute the failings of the welfare state to a variety of technical, administrative factors. Titmuss attributed the failure of the welfare state to abolish poverty and reduce inequality to factors such as the lack of tools to monitor the effects of social change and the overall impact of the expansion of public and private services,[94] or to failure on the part of the governments to grasp the complexity of the problems of deprivation and to appreciate the difficulties of reaching poor and minority groups and of getting them to use universal services.[95] Crosland added two further, similar explanations. The first was a lack of clarity about service objectives and, as a result, too little effort to coordinate policies, particularly in deprived inner city areas.[96] The second explanation was the failure of successive governments to achieve economic growth. Crosland often reiterated the view that a stagnant economy meant a stagnant public welfare system and an end to further redistribution.

The economic recession and the cuts in social services introduced by the Conservative governments in the 1980s have brought forth more structural explanations from Fabians. Townsend explains the existence of widespread poverty in contemporary Britain within a theoretical framework 'rooted in class relations' and concludes that 'if poverty is to be reduced, there must be less differentiation hierarchically of the employed population *and* a small proportionate share of total national resources by higher income groups'.[97] Walker's discussion of the need for a new social strategy takes an equally structural view of the failure of social policies and calls for thorough-going changes in education, social security and other services.[98] Similarly, Meacher's analysis of the distribution of power in society leads him to structural explanations for the failure of both the economy and of egalitarian measures.[99]

How do the Fabians then see the relationship between the welfare state and socialism? From the very beginning it was realised that the social service state is different from a socialist society. Tawney, Titmuss and Crosland agreed that the welfare state is not socialism even though they disagreed on some of the essential features of a socialist society. There was a great deal of optimism, however, that the welfare state would act as an important influence for socialist change. The public would soon come to realise that the benefits conferred by the welfare state were only a foretaste of an even better life under socialism. Social services were seen as having a central role to play in this change of public attitudes. 'By changing the lives of individuals and opening new possibilities to them', wrote Tawney, 'they change social psychology. The altered psychology acts as a permanent force modifying social structure which, in turn, as it is transformed, sets minds and wills at work to insist on further modifications.'[100]

Today there is greater scepticism among Fabians about the effects of social services on people's consciousness. It is people's economic interests that shape their attitudes towards the social services rather than the other way round. This has brought about the realisation that the welfare state may be a staging post towards socialism but the road is longer and more difficult than anticipated in the past and there are no historical imperatives that lead inexorably from the welfare state to socialism.

In brief, while Fabian socialists see the welfare state as only the limited and partial achievement of some socialist goals, they remain modestly optimistic about its influence. They see it not as dampening down the political forces making for further social change but rather as providing some of the dynamic necessary for such change. The welfare state is still seen as an unstable compromise and a potential stepping stone toward socialism. It is now more widely and openly acknowledged by Fabians, however, that whether the contemporary welfare state develops into a socialist society or remains as it is, or regresses to a residual form of welfare state, depends on the balance of economic and political forces in the country.

5

The Marxists

In spite of their diametrically opposed views on social values, the nature of the state, the role of government and the desirability of the welfare state, anti-collectivists and Marxists share two common characteristics in their approach to these issues. First, they examine them within developed theoretical frameworks to a greater extent than the other two groups of thinkers. Second, they adhere to basic principles rather than to pragmatic incrementalism in the proposals they put forward for reforming the welfare state despite the public hostility that this approach arouses. Hayek expressed this rejection of incrementalism in 1949 when he wrote:

> To advocate any clear-cut principles of social order is today an almost certain way to incur the stigma of being an unpractical doctrinaire. It has come to be regarded as the sign of the judicious mind that in social matters one does not adhere to fixed principles but decides each question 'on its merits'; that one is generally guided by expediency and is ready to compromise between opposed views.[1]

Marxists have a great deal of sympathy with this view for, if anything, their ideas have been even more stigmatised than those of anti-collectivists who, as we saw in Chapter 2, have recently gained greater respectability.

Social values

Marx's writings are a relentless critique of the inhumanity of the capitalist system as it existed during his lifetime. Working-class people were exploited and they became alienated from their fellow workers and from their true selves. But one finds very little in Marx's or Engels's writings about the type of values that they would have liked to see governing social relations in a socialist or communist society. This was due partly to their belief that it would be Utopian to prescribe such values in advance and partly due to their materialistic interpretation of change in history which is discussed in the following section. Suffice it to say here that they saw social values as the result of the prevailing economic conditions in society and believed that a change in values in a socialist society would come about as a result of the social ownership of the means of production and distribution. In the same way that under capitalism the dominant ideology is congruent with the capitalist form of production and distribution which favours the few, under socialism the reigning ideology would reflect the socialist form of production and distribution which served the interests of all alike.

Marx and Engels allowed themselves, however, the luxury of making some sketchy comments on the broad principles which should govern the distribution of income and the freedom of the individual in society. During the stage following the overthrow or transformation of an advanced capitalist system – the socialist stage – the guiding distributive principle will be 'From each according to his abilities, to each according to his work'. During the later, more advanced stage – the communist stage – the principle would change to 'From each according to his abilities, to each according to his needs'.[2] Marx was aware that distributive principles could only have any practical meaning if they reflected the prevailing economic conditions and through these public attitudes. Thus, only during the communist stage could distribution be according to need because only then would there be abundance of material goods and only then would people's consciousness have changed from individualism and competitiveness to collectivism and altruism.

Miliband writes of 'a fundamental distinction' which Marx made between 'political emancipation' and 'human emancipation'. The former included civic rights such as the extension of the suffrage, representative institutions and the curbing of arbitrary power, and was attainable within the capitalist system. In contrast, 'human emancipation' cannot be achieved simply through political changes but depends upon the revolutionary transformation of the economic and social order.[3] Capitalism cannot create a truly human environment. It cannot provide the economic and social conditions for men and women to realise their true potentialities. This 'human emancipation' would be accompanied by a liberation of human personality from the enslaving pressures of the capitalist division of labour. This is an even more difficult concept than the notion of distribution according to need. The most graphic illustration occurs in the following description by Marx of a communist society:

> where nobody has one exclusive sphere of activity but each can become accomplished in any branch he wishes, society regulates the general production and thus makes it possible for me to do one thing today and another tomorrow, to hunt in the morning, fish in the afternoon, raise cattle in the evening, criticise after dinner, just as I have a mind without ever becoming a hunter, fisherman, shepherd or critic.[4]

Marxists see individual freedom in much broader terms than the anti-collectivists. They see it in terms of the removal of obstacles to human emancipation and self-realisation – something which can only be achieved by collective action. Like the Fabians, they see liberty and equality not only as compatible with each other but also as mutually enriching. By implication, Laski saw three conditions as necessary for the realisation of liberty in society. First, he argued that liberty can never exist 'in the presence of special privilege'.[5] Second, 'where the rights of some depend upon the pleasures of others'[6] and third, where the incidence of state action is biased in favour of one group as it manifestly is under capitalism. He is arguing in effect that liberty in the Marxist sense cannot be fully implemented for the mass of the people in a capitalist society.

Strachey too took this view of liberty. Civil liberties under capitalism, important though they are, for the mass of the workers are 'poor, thin and half-illusory things'.[7] The task of Marxist politics is, in Miliband's words, 'to defend these freedoms: and to make possible their extension and enlargement of the removal of their class boundaries'.[8] If this is to be achieved, bourgeois freedoms must be complemented with economic liberties – employment opportunities, good wages and promotion prospects. Liberty and equality must, therefore, be seen as parts of a whole. The absence of equality in either the political or the economic field produces inequality in the other – a view expressed by Laski when he argued that: 'Political equality . . . is never real unless it is accompanied by virtual economic equality; political power, otherwise, is bound to be the handmaid of economic power.'[9]

But what is equality? Strachey follows Marx closely and distinguishes between distribution according to 'the quality of work done' under socialism and distribution according to individual need under communism. He warns, however, that distribution according to individual need necessitates not only general economic affluence but also a different value system. The changing of values, he feels, is a much more difficult proposition than the achievement of affluence.[10] Laski rejects the charge that Marxists view equality as sameness. In its broad sense equality means first 'the absence of special privilege' and second that 'adequate opportunities are laid open to all'.[11] Differences are compatible with egalitarianism provided that 'such differences as exist must not be differences inexplicable in terms of reason. Distinctions of wealth or status must be distinctions to which all men can attain and they must be required by the common welfare.'[12] He also rejects the specific idea that economic equality means equal incomes for all – for three reasons: first, 'that there seems no justice in an equal reward for unequal effort'; second, it does not 'seem just to reward equally where needs are unequal'; and third, complete income equality is contrary to 'the mental habits of western civilisation' with the result that it will be impossible for governments to enforce.[13]

Laski also rejects, though with some reluctance, Marx's view of distribution according to individual need. He approves of the principle but rejects it because in practice it would be unworkable. He points out that individual need is difficult to define and so governments have no option but to use the notion of average need for policy purposes.[14] He therefore adopts the notion of relative equality. In practical terms, this means first that 'every need related to the civic minimum, every need, that is, which, when unsatisfied, prevents the attainment of effective citizenship must be satisfied before we deal with needs above the civic minimum'.[15] Second, after the satisfaction of basic needs, differences in reward 'would be built either upon effort or ability'[16] to take account of the varying contributions of individuals in different occupations. It is a view that is very similar indeed to that of Tawney discussed in the previous chapter.

Society and the state

Like all other political philosophies, Marxism is both a form of political commitment and a social theory attempting to provide an explanation of how society functions. It is, perhaps, the most detailed attempt to articulate the forces that shape societies and their institutions, including the social services.

In general, contemporary Marxists agree with the materialist explanation of history, of change and stability in society, put forward by Marx and Engels even though there are substantial differences of opinion on how this process actually works out in practice. According to this view, in every society the economic structure is

> the real foundation, on which rise legal and political super-structures and to which correspond definite forms of social consciousness. The mode of production in material life determines the general character of the social, political and spiritual processes of life. It is not the consciousness of men that determines their existence but, on the contrary, their social existence determines their consciousness.[17]

In other words, the way society earns its living accounts for the prevailing political system, educational system, the nature of art and music, of ideology, and so on. Similarly, the nature of a person's job has crucial implications for his general life-style and way of thinking.

This division of society into structure and superstructure has clear implications for those seeking change in society. Both Marx and Engels, however, were anxious to point out that there is a great deal of debate on how the economic structure affects parts of the superstructure. Marx acknowledged that the superstructure of any society is more complex than its economic base partly because it involves the actions of classes, groups and individuals and partly because, being the outcome of historical change, it always tends to include elements of the past that may not be fully congruent with the current economic base of society. Indeed, in an attempt to answer their critics, Engels qualified the importance of economic factors to the point of relative insignificance:

> according to the materialist conception of history, the deter-mining element in history is, *ultimately*, the production and

reproduction in real life. More than this neither Marx nor I have ever asserted. If, therefore, somebody twists this into the statement that the economic element is the *only* determining one, he transforms it into a meaningless, abstract and absurd phrase. The economic situation is the basis but the various elements of the superstructure . . . also exercise their influence upon the course of the historical struggles and in many cases preponderate in determining their *form*.[18]

Thus, the Marxist conception of history and change can be seen either as economic determinism, or as a less rigid doctrine, but with economic factors usually being seen as the most significant. It is this latter view which seems to have gained acceptance among writers about politics and the welfare state. Thus Laski, while stressing that economic changes are paramount, acknowledged that other factors are also important though the part they play 'depends upon an environment, the nature of which is determined by its system of economic relationships'.[19] Miliband takes a similar view when he rejects economic determinism and accepts the view that the economic base must be used as 'a *starting-point*, as a matter of the *first instance*' against which changes in the superstructure must be examined.[20] The obvious tension in the materialist conception of history is that rigid economic determinism can become a strait-jacket rendering politics, education, religion, etc., irrelevant while relative economic determinism can become a form of pluralism attributing equal weight to politics, education, religion, etc. Somewhere between these two extreme positions lies the favoured standpoint of most Marxist writers today. Whatever the standpoint, however, the materialist conception of history must always remain unproven because even though one can acknowledge the importance of the economic structure, the difficulty, as Raymond Williams has pointed out, 'lies in estimating the final importance of a factor which never, in practice, appears in isolation'.[21] It follows from a materialistic perception of history that the relationship of different groups in society to the means of production is what determines the differential power of these groups and their relationship with one another. In a capitalist society the means of production are owned and managed by a small minority who thus enjoy most of the wealth created by the production system. The majority of the population do not have any share in the ownership of the means of production and they have, therefore, to rely for their livelihood on their labour. Thus the two main classes – the capitalist class and the working class –

are locked in a structurally antagonistic relationship and hence are in fundamental conflict with each other. Class conflict is, therefore, endemic in a capitalist system and it can only be abolished by the abolition of the private ownership of the means of production, that is of the capitalist system itself. Class conflict may take different forms and it can be at high or low levels but it can never be abolished in a capitalist society.

Class conflict takes place in the economic, political and cultural sectors and it assumes several forms, ranging from the very violent to the urbane and peaceful. As Taylor-Gooby and Dale put it, 'when we speak of class struggle we are generally referring to the myriads of ways in which the exploited class struggles against the power of those who own/control the means of production'.[22] Thus, protests and demonstrations, both peaceful and violent, wage negotiations and strikes, voting at parliamentary and local elections, political debates, and so on are all part and parcel of the ongoing class conflict that is inherent in a capitalist society. Defined in these broad terms, class conflict is not amenable to quantification and, therefore, any statements about trends in the volume of class conflict over the years carry little weight.

Marx and Engels clearly recognised the existence of conflicts other than class conflict. What they sought to emphasise, however, was that conflict between wage earners and capitalists is the primary type of conflict in capitalist society. The distinction between class conflict and conflict between racial, religious and interest groups is that these latter types of conflict can be resolved within the capitalist system itself. In Laski's words: 'The distinction, which is ultimate, between all other social antagonisms and that between capital and labour is that the resolution of the latter can be achieved only by an alteration of the legal postulates of capitalist society.'[23] Marxists also acknowledge the contribution which individual political figures can make to the course of events in a country but they see such contributions as being moulded and constrained by the broad economic and political environment in which they operate. In Marx's often-quoted sentence: 'Men make their own history, but they do not make it just as they please; they do not make it under circumstances chosen by themselves but under circumstances directly uncountered, given and transmitted from the past.'[24]

In brief, class conflict is not the only vehicle for change in a capitalist society but it is the most important. Inevitably, there are differences of opinion among Marxists about the relative importance of such other factors and about their relationship to class conflict. Marxists, however, are united in their belief that class conflict will sooner or later lead to the overthrow of the capitalist system in advanced capitalist societies. As capitalism develops both the internal contradictions of capitalism deepen and the strength of the working class grows. It is for this reason that Marx and Engels saw the socialist transformation coming about only in advanced capitalist societies and not in economically underdeveloped capitalist societies. 'No social order', Marx wrote, 'ever perishes before all the productive forces for which there is room in it have developed; and new, higher relations of production never appear before the material conditions of their existence have matured in the womb of the old society itself.'[25]

The final change could come about either peacefully or violently depending on the balance of class forces prevailing in society. Marx's general trend of argument, however, was that in most countries the road to socialism would be through non-peaceful means because of the natural refusal of the capitalist class to give up its privileges peacefully. He acknowledged, however, that 'there are countries, such as America and England . . . where the workers may attain their goal by peaceful means'.[26] Engels, who outlived Marx by many years and witnessed the growth of working-class movements leading to economic, political and social reform, was more hopeful than Marx about the peaceful road to socialism.

British Marxist writers have shown a marked reluctance to approve of violence for political ends even as a last resort. They recognise that violence by the working class may turn out to be counterproductive as it is bound to bring forth a violent counteraction by the capitalist class. Moreover, they consider the peaceful road to socialism as superior to a violent one for, though it is bound to be a slow process, it will create a truly socialist society based on the consent of the majority. Thus Laski, in spite of understandable hesitations, retained his faith in constitutional government in Britain – a position shared by many Marxists.

> Where the members of a state enjoy fundamental political rights in a degree real enough to make effectively possible the transformation of dissent into orthodoxy, I believe that it is the duty of the citizen to exhaust the means placed at his disposal by the constitution of the state before resorting to revolution. I admit that the nature of capitalist democracy weights the scales unduly against him. I admit, also, that this is a counsel of prudent expediency rather than an ultimate moral right. But I believe that the gains which are inherent in the techniques of

constitutionalism are profounder, even though they are slower, than those which are implicit in the revolutionary alternative.[27]

During the post-war years, there has been an even greater rejection of the idea of using violence for political ends. The British Communist Party was the first in Western Europe to accept the parliamentary road to socialism in 1951. Other European communist parties followed so that today the 'reformist' road to socialism is the general policy of the Euro-Communist movement.

As was pointed out in the previous chapters, Fabians emphasise that the only road to socialism is through gradualist reform. Though there is a degree of similarity between the Fabian and the Marxist approaches, there are three main differences between them. The Marxist perception includes both parliamentary and extra-parliamentary struggles – 'for instance, industrial struggles, strikes, sit-ins, work-ins, demonstrations, marches, campaigns, etc., designed to advance specific or general demands, oppose governmental policies, protest against given measures, and so on'.[28] The Fabians are, in theory, against extra-parliamentary activities though they approve of some varieties in certain circumstances. Secondly, reformism to the Marxists, unlike the Fabians and others, is only legitimate as part of a coherent strategy for the socialist transformation of society. Many Fabians, however, also view reforms in this way – as changes desirable in themselves and as means to the broader aim of the gradual creation of a socialist society. The third difference between Marxist and Fabian attitudes to the reformist approach to societal change is the Marxist anxieties about such an approach. Fabians see it as the only way forward; Marxists see it as a possible strategy but one beset by difficulties. It can lead to accommodation to the *status quo*. It can lead to the incorporation of the working class into a cosier relationship with its capitalist masters. It is threatened by 'the seemingly inexorable propensity of reformist parties to slide from a commitment to socialism towards the less arduous pursuit of social reforms'.[29]

The recent increased Marxist faith in 'reformism' is largely the result of the realisation that working-class people in advanced industrial societies have no appetite for revolutionary change and the fact that it now seems less likely that the capitalist class will attempt actively to overthrow a left-wing government pursuing radical policies. What is more likely to happen in such a situation is that the capitalist class will attempt to create the maximum possible economic disruption, usually in alliance with the international agencies of capital.

Whatever the future may hold, the fact remains that no advanced capitalist society has yet been transformed into a socialist society contrary to Marx's and Engels's anticipation that such transformations were imminent in many countries. Why? Two inter-related forces are said to have prevented the working class from using its vast numerical superiority to alter the socio-economic system to its advantage: the economic power of the capitalist class and the nature of the state.

Advanced capitalism has seen the growth of large national and international private companies whose influence over the economy of a country is always very strong and, at times, crucial. Many non-Marxists share Miliband's view that advanced capitalism is 'all but synonymous with giant enterprise and nothing about the economic organisations of these countries is more basically important than the increasing domination of key sectors of their industrial, financial and commercial life by a relatively small number of giant firms often interlinked'.[30] Decisions by these large companies on whether to invest, where to invest, whether to raise prices, whether and when to withdraw capital from a country cannot but influence government policies to the benefit of capitalism. Labour and social democratic governments will have to be just as deferential to the power of such companies as Conservative governments.

Marxists insist that the managerial revolution has had no fundamental effect on either the concentration of economic power or on the paramountcy of profit in economic operations. Management may well conduct the affairs of large corporations with additional aims in mind apart from profit maximisation, but there is no denying, claim Baran and Sweezy, that 'profits, even though not the ultimate goal, are the necessary means to all ultimate goals. As such, they become the immediate, unique, unifying quantitative aim of corporate policies, the touchstone of corporate rationality, the measure of corporate success.'[31] The 'soulful' corporation has not replaced the 'soulless' corporation as the exponents of the managerial revolution thesis claim. Nor has the power of the managers overridden the power of the owners of wealth. There may occasionally be differences of opinion and interest between these two overlapping groups but 'the differences of purpose and motivation which may exist between them are overshadowed by a basic community of interests'.[32] In summary, the concentration and internationalisation of capital has strengthened the influence which the capitalist class has always had over governments, including those with socialist intentions.

No other concept in the Marxist vocabulary has received so much attention during the past decade as that of the state. It is neither necessary nor possible to examine the debate at length here. Instead, only those aspects which are relevant to the present discussion will be touched upon. In the writings of Marx and Engels, three distinct forms of the state can be found, each representing a different view of the balance of class forces in society. The first variant is the classic view of the state first expressed by Marx and Engels in the Communist Manifesto where they concluded that: 'The executive of the modern state is but a committee for managing the common affairs of the whole bourgeoisie.' Miliband describes this as 'the core proposition of Marxism on the subject of the state'.[33] In other words, government policies, as well as the absence of such policies, serve the interests of the capitalist class and strengthen its position in society. The state is seen simply as an instrument of class domination. Most, but by no means all, Marxists today accept that this form of the state cannot be said to exist in advanced capitalist societies where both parties of the left and trade unions exercise so much political and industrial power.

The second variant of the state is what may be called the 'temporarily autonomous' state. 'By way of exception, however', wrote Engels, 'periods occur in which the warring classes balance each other so nearly that the state power, as ostensible mediator, acquires for the moment a certain degree of independence of both.'[34] In other words, this form of the state exists in the very exceptional circumstances when both the capitalist and the working class are too weak to exercise any strong influence on state apparatuses or when there is a balance of power between them. In such circumstances, the state derives its power from the control of government positions and it serves the interests of its personnel. Again, most Marxists agree that such a conception of the state does not fit with the power realities of advanced capitalist societies.

The third view of the state, and the one which commands most support among Marxists today, is the 'relative autonomy' thesis. According to this view, though the state tends to serve the interests of the capitalist class, it also supports policies which can be contrary to these interests. It does this either because of political pressure from the working class or as a result of deliberate decisions by governments to provide services beneficial to the working class in order to undermine radicalist tendencies in it. There is also the possibility of the state providing services which are contrary to the interests of some sections of the capitalist class but are helpful to the long-term interests of capital in general. Miliband argues that Marx and Engels attributed a considerable degree of autonomy to the state. Their statement that the task of the state was to manage 'the *common* affairs of the *whole* bourgeoisie' suggests a bourgeoisie composed of different elements with separate and specific interests as well as common ones, and that it is the state which must manage its common affairs. To do this it must have a degree of autonomy.[35] In these ways the state serves the interests of the capitalist class in the long-term even though it may be forced, or decide for itself, to make concessions to the working class from time to time.

In spite of heated discussions among Marxists, there is agreement that there are four main reasons why the state serves the interests of the capitalist class. First, the top personnel of the state apparatus come from the same socio-economic background as the top personnel of industry and the mass media. The result is that although there is no absolute unanimity of views between these groups, they, nevertheless, in Miliband's words, share 'a cluster of common ideological and political positions and attitudes, common values and perspectives' which are favourable to the capitalist form of production and distribution.[36] Second, the economic power of the capitalist class enables it to exert such influence on governments directly and indirectly. Third, the capitalist mode of production inevitably imposes certain structural constraints and any government. 'A capitalist economy has its own "rationality" to which government and state must sooner or later submit, and usually sooner.'[37] Fourth, the market institutions of capitalism generate attitudes and values which predispose democratic states to serve the interests of capital. Thus, even left-wing governments see it as their duty to provide the conditions required for the capitalist economy to grow, even if it means that living standards of working class people have to suffer for a while.

The view of the state one adopts has crucial implications for such important and related issues as the possibilities of the parliamentary road to socialism, the use of violence, and the value of reforms. Thus it is no surprise that the upsurge of support for the 'relative autonomy' thesis has coincided with the growth of the Euro-Communist movement favouring the parliamentary road to socialism. The question, however, of just how relative the autonomy of the state is remains unresolved for, as Mishra has pointed out, the limits of this autonomy 'cannot be laid down by any theory'.[38] It therefore remains a matter of personal interpretation among Marxists as to how free the state is to pursue policies that are detrimental to the interests of the capitalist class.

It is implied in what has been said so far that class power and state power, separately and together, have used a variety of methods to maintain the capitalist order. These can be grouped under three headings: economic, repressive and ideological. The subordinate position of workers in the labour market – the fact that they have to rely on their labour for their livelihood, their inability to control security of employment, and so on – means that they may reluctantly tolerate the existing economic system even though they have no ideological commitment to it. The disciplinary role of paid employment increases at times of high unemployment and decreases, but never disappears, at times of full employment. The repressive methods that used to be so common in the early days of capitalism have weakened but they still exist in a modified form and they are resorted to very occasionally in welfare capitalist societies. Increasingly, the state in welfare capitalism uses ideological forms of control – the propagation of the dominant ideology through the official agencies of the state and the informal processes of society.[39] Gramsci, for example, emphasised the major role of the state in the organisation of consent and legitimation. In the light of these insights, Marxists are increasingly recognising the importance of the theoretical, ideological struggle. As Barnett put it, 'until a majority of the working class actively *desire socialism*, they will continue to be willing to accept bourgeois solutions to the recurrent crises of capitalism, however temporarily acute'.[40]

The role of government

It follows from what has been said so far that Marxists favour both a substantial extension of government activity in the economic and the social field and a move towards a more participative and democratic system. This section concentrates on the economic role of government because social welfare is discussed in more detail in the following section. The traditional economic strategy of Marxists has consisted of two main programmes: nationalisation of the means of production and distribution and industrial democracy at work.

Nationalisation is justified on both political and economic considerations. The private ownership of the means of production clearly involves the concentration of economic power in the hands of the capitalist class. This, in turn, means that political power, too, is concentrated in the same class because, as Strachey put it, 'political power and economic power are, in the last resort, merely aspects of one indivisible whole, namely power itself'.[41] The growth of national and international companies has added strength to the nationalisation argument for such companies are more powerful and less amenable to government control than small enterprises. Holland shows that the concentration of economic power has been substantial in Britain during the post-war period. While the top one hundred manufacturing firms controlled only 15 per cent of net manufacturing output in 1910 and only a mere 20 per cent in 1950, by 1970 the corresponding proportion was 46 per cent and by 1985 it is projected to reach 66 per cent.[42]

The claim that concentration of economic power inevitably means concentration of political power is acknowledged by many non-Marxists – of whom Galbraith and Lindblom are the best known examples. Lindblom expresses this duality of power as follows.

> Because public functions in the market system rest in the hands of businessmen, it follows that jobs, prices, production, growth, the standard of living, and the economic security of everyone all rest in their hands. Consequently, government officials cannot be indifferent to how well business performs its functions. Depression, inflation, or other economic disasters can bring down a government. A major function of government, therefore, is to see to it that businessmen perform their tasks.[43]

The economic arguments for nationalising private enterprises are as strong as the political arguments. It is considered immoral that though profits are produced through the labour of the workers, they are reaped by the large shareholders who do not have to work. Under such conditions, workers feel alienated from the work process with the result that not only do they themselves suffer psychologically but economic production suffers as well.

It is increasingly acknowledged, however, that nationalisation measures cannot by themselves create a socialist society though they are seen as a necessary prerequisite. As Miliband concludes, nationalisation 'cannot by itself resolve all the problems associated with industrial society. What it can do, however, is to remove the greatest of all barriers to their solution and at least create the basis for the creation of a rational and humane social order.'[44]

There is now general acceptance among Marxists that national-ised industries in a socialist society will be democratically run with maximum workers' participation. This is not a new idea for Engels insisted that without such participation, nationalisation could not be part of a socialist way of life. He pointed out that if nationalisation by itself constituted socialism, 'Napoleon and Metternich would rank among the founders of socialism'.[45] The experience of nationalised, non-participatory industry in Eastern Europe has given new force to Engels and Marx's insistence on socialist participation. Thus recent editions of the policy docu-ment of the British Communist Party, *The British Road to Socialism*, lay increasing stress on all forms of participation and the democratisation of industrial and public life.[46]

The benefits claimed for industrial democracy are many and varied and they have not changed much over the years: it extends and gives real meaning to political democracy; it reduces industrial conflict and promotes industrial cooperation; it en-hances individual satisfaction with work; it increases productivity and hence the standard of living of all in society. There has, as yet, been very little hard discussion of the possible problems involved in industrial democracy programmes particularly its possible ill-effects on efficiency and productivity.

The nationalisation and socialisation of the means of produc-tion would obviously make it easier for governments to plan both their economic and social policies. Government planning with the widest form of public participation is essential for democracy and socialism. Laski's insistence that parliamentary democracy is desirable and compatible with a socialist planned society has now been generally accepted by the communist parties of Western Europe as well as by many prominent Marxists. It is in marked contrast to the Leninist, let alone the Stalinist, approach to socialism. It is rather in line with Rosa Luxemburg's firm belief in parliamentary democracy and socialism: 'Without general elections', she wrote, 'without unrestricted freedom of press and assembly, without a free struggle of opinion, life dies out in every public institution, becomes a mere semblance of life in which only the bureaucracy remains as the active element.'[47] Neverthe-less, the suppression of parliamentary democracy in Eastern European countries, which are referred to as 'socialist' by many commentators, has created a crisis for many Marxists. On one hand they proclaim their faith in parliamentary democracy and on the other they are identified by the media as supporters of the East European regimes. The emphasis on parliamentary democracy among many contemporary Marxists is, however, unmistakable despite media and other claims to the contrary. Poulantzas summed up his belief in representative democratic institutions in a socialist society as follows: 'But one thing is certain – socialism will be democratic or it will not be at all.'[48] However, until a country with a Marxist government can prove that democracy and Marxist socialism can co-exist, Marxism will continue to be identified with dictatorship in the minds of the public in Western European and other advanced capitalist societies.

The welfare state

In this section three separate but related issues are discussed: the reasons given by Marxists for the introduction of social policy measures by governments; the roles and functions of social policies under welfare capitalism; and the Marxist view of socialist social policies.

In the Marxist literature three main explanations have been offered for the growth of social policy: class conflict, the Machiavellianism of the capitalist class, and the requirements of the capitalist system for increased efficiency. The class conflict view has its origins in Marx's discussion of factory legislation in Britain. The main driving force behind factory legislation was, according to Marx, the workers' newly found industrial and political power. He acknowledged that other groups in society – the landed aristocracy and philanthropic individuals – supported factory reforms but saw these as secondary to the power of the working class. 'The creation of a normal working day', he wrote, 'is, therefore, the product of a protracted civil war, more or less dissembled between the capitalist class and the working class.'[49] Laski in the 1930s adopted a rather different approach to Marx when he wrote:

> Social legislation is not the outcome of a rational and objective willing of the common good by all members of the community alike; it is the price paid for those legal principles which secure the predominance of the owners of property. It waxes and wanes in terms of their prosperity. It is the body of concessions offered to avert a decisive challenge to the principles by which their authority is maintained.[50]

There are, in Laski's view, clear elements of a belief in the Machiavellianism of the capitalist class. The government as representative of the interests of the capitalist class makes tactical concessions to the working class to forestall a direct challenge to the existing order. It has its classical example in the social insurance reforms introduced by Bismarck in Germany at the turn of the last century.

The reason why these two views are difficult to separate is that it is almost impossible to know whether reforms are squeezed out of the government by working-class pressure or whether they are granted freely but with an ulterior motive in mind. This ambiguity is often found in the work of Marxist writers who support these two explanations. Thus, Miliband sees the extension of the social services at the end of the last war in Britain as 'part of the "ransom" the working class had been able to extract from their rulers in the course of a hundred years'.[51] The word 'extract' implies that the development was forced on the capitalist class by working class pressure but it could also mean that services were offered as 'ransom'. To all intents and purposes, therefore, the class conflict and the Machiavellianism thesis are best explored together as two aspects of one explanation.

The extent and types of reform the capitalist class will concede will depend on the dynamics of the particular situation in which the class conflict takes place. The unity and consciousness and hence the relative strength of the working class is the first obvious variable in this equation. It is no coincidence that most of the important social reforms have been attained since the working class won the right to vote. Another important variable is the actual timing of working-class pressures for reform. Thus war time and the immediate aftermath of war have proved very fertile reform periods. The state of the economy is another relevant consideration. The capitalist class can better afford to make concessions to the working-class demands at times of prosperity. At times of recession, this obviously becomes more difficult. The final factor is, of course, the nature of working-class demands. Marxists point out that the nature of the dominant ideology acts in such a way as to moderate the demands made by working-class groups. Even so, such demands will obviously be resisted and contained as far as possible.

During the last decade, the class conflict explanation has been complemented, absorbed or even replaced, depending on the particular Marxist writer, by 'the requirements of the capitalist system' explanation. This model has its origins in Marx's views that, if left to itself, the capitalist system of production and distribution has an inherent tendency towards stagnation, under-consumption, a falling rate of profit and periodic crises. The state is forced to intervene to enable the capitalist system to overcome these recurrent tendencies and to increase its efficiency. In other words, public and social expenditure develop and expand primarily because they benefit the capitalist system. Though the capitalist state has always been interventionist, its activities expanded tremendously after the acceptance of Keynesian theories of economic management and the ascendancy of monopoly capitalism with its ability easily to extract government aid in kind or in cash.

At its most extreme, this explanation assumes a functionalist character that is similar to the Parsonian functionalist explanation except that the latter sees government services as serving the interests of all. Basically, however, they are both system integration theories of government services. Mandel tends to see the growth of all government services – economic and social – as the result of the functional needs of advanced capitalism as opposed to the situation obtaining in the early *laissez-faire* period when only minimal government aid was necessary.[52] Baran and Sweezy, in their study of the growth of American capitalism, adopt a similar perspective – seeing the *laissez-faire* stage of capitalism when substantial government services were not crucial to capitalism as a passing phase to be succeeded by advanced, monopoly capitalism which is inherently dependent on govern-ment services.[53] The main weakness of these rigidly functionalist explanations is that they are not explanations in the sense of being amenable to empirical investigation, let alone testing. Writers who confine their attention to the growth of social services rather than public expenditure in general tend to adopt perspectives which attempt to combine the class conflict and the needs of capital explanations. Such attempts, however, have not been very successful with the result that they lean more towards one or other of these two explanations. Ginsburg, for example, insists that: 'the welfare state is not considered here as an untrammelled achievement of the working class struggle. . . . Nor is it viewed as an institution shaped largely by the demands and requirements of the capitalist economy.' It is rather the result of the interplay of these factors in 'specific historical contexts'.[54] When, however, he applies this explanation to the growth of social security and housing he tends to give more emphasis to the benefits accruing to capital than to labour. One cannot help but ask: 'If this is the case why are Conservative governments today cutting down on these services and why are trade unions objecting?'

Gough, too, attempts to combine the two explanations:

> We have discerned two factors of importance in explaining the growth of the welfare state: the degree of class conflict and, especially, the strength and form of working-class struggle, and the ability of the capitalist state to formulate and implement policies to secure the long-term reproduction of capitalist social relations.[55]

He argues that neither explanation is adequate by itself to explain all types of reforms at all times. But he concludes that 'it is the threat of a powerful working-class movement which galvanises the ruling class to think more cohesively and strategically'[56] and thus introduce social policy reforms. It is clearly difficult to combine these two explanations effectively because one adopts an action frame of reference while the other is a static form of analysis. They also have different implications for the next point of our discussion.

What of the Marxist view of the role and functions of social policies under welfare capitalism? In both the Marxist and the non-Marxist literature, there has been a tendency to assume that an analysis of the development of social policies was also a contribution to an understanding of their functions. This may or may not be so. A policy may be introduced as the result of a protracted working-class struggle, but it cannot therefore be assumed without further exploration that it gives most benefit to the working class.

Nevertheless, by rooting and grounding analysis of the development of social policy in a broader social analysis, Marxism does open the way to a deeper understanding of the varied roles and functions of social policies in capitalist society. If social services are to be found in all advanced capitalist societies, and if they are the product of the conflicting pulls and pushes of class conflict, capitalist Machiavellianism and the requirements of the capitalist system, then their functions are complex, if not contradictory.

O'Connor's work makes a valuable contribution in this area because this focus is directly on the functions of public policy in advanced capitalist societies. The capitalist state, he argues, 'must try to fulfil two basic and often mutually contradictory functions – accumulation and legitimation'.[57] The state must, in other words, enable private capital to remain profitable but it must also provide legitimation for the existing economic and social order. All public expenditure has these two functions though O'Connor divides it into three categories: social investment such as government aid to industry or transport services; social consumption such as education, health and housing, which lowers the reproduction cost of labour and hence increases profitability; and social expenses such as social security benefits, the police and social work, which promote and maintain social harmony.

O'Connor goes on to argue that these functions are contradictory and that they create a fiscal crisis for the capitalist state because of the increasing difficulties involved in raising the revenue required to meet the cost of public services. At the same time, the state cannot afford to neglect them because of the effects such neglect would have on profitability and social harmony. As Gough puts it: 'The welfare state is a product of the *contradictory* development of capitalist society and in turn has generated new contradictions which every day become more apparent.'[58]

O'Connor's analysis is supported by many Marxists including Offe who neatly sums up the state's dilemma. 'The contradiction is that while capitalism cannot co-exist *with* the welfare state, neither can it exist *without* the welfare state.'[59] Offe goes further to show that what is implied in O'Connor's work is that the welfare state can act as a destabilising force despite its avowed aim of promoting social harmony. It does this by the effects it can have, for example, on rates of taxation, work incentives and rates of profit – an argument that is not too dissimilar to that made by several anti-collectivists.

O'Connor's work has proved immensely stimulating in its analysis of the functions of state expenditure and its assessment of their contradictions. It has, however, three weaknesses relevant to our discussion. The first is that he fails to distinguish between the formal, intended functions of public policy and the informal, unintended consequences. The second is that O'Connor's rather abstract categorisation of the functions of public expenditure underestimates the very real benefits derived by working-class people from public services. Third, it grossly underestimates, as we shall see in the next chapter, the contribution which economic growth can make to political stability. Thus services which promote 'accumulation' are at the same time promoting 'legitimation'.

Simple class conflict explanations of the development of social policy imply that all developments are potential gains for the working class. The realisation that the factors shaping policy develoment are more complex awakens doubts as to whether the workers will always be the sole or even the main beneficiaries of expanding welfare expenditure. Critical analysis of the functions and role of social policies in capitalist society gives such doubts support and substanace. For these and other reasons – for example doubts about reformist policies generally – many Marxists are today ambivalent about the importance of social reform to the working class and lack the original enthusiasm of Marx or Engels.

In this last section the sparse and brief comments – general and specific – by Marxists on what makes social policies socialist will be examined. The discussion is difficult not only because of the sparsity of evidence but also because of the distinction between socialism and communism. It is not always clear whether Marxist comments on socialist social policies refer to the socialist stage or the communist stage.

Marx and Engels envisaged that an increasing proportion of a country's income would be set aside for the satisfaction of 'communal needs' as the country proceeded through the socialist stage until it reached the communist stage when provision of services would be based totally on individual need. Their comments on individual social services were tantalisingly brief but it is nevertheless worth discussing and comparing them with the views of contemporary Marxists.

In the case of education, Marx and Engels's comments add up to an educational system under socialism that would be 'universal, secular, polytechnical, participatory and environmentalist'.[60] It is not clear whether by universal they meant free of charge and open to all at all stages or whether they meant free of charge at all stages but selective at the university level, or some other form of combination. Their emphasis on secular education was designed to counteract the rather heavy moralistic teaching that tended to accompany religious teaching in schools in their day. Polytechnical education was the quality of socialist education they stressed most. Marx felt that a polytechnical system of education combined academic and industrial training and it would not only stimulate economic growth but it was 'the only method of producing fully developed human beings'.[61] The latter phrase denotes Marx and Engels's view that men and women in socialist societies should be able to perform many occupational tasks in order to do away with the division of labour as well as the distinction between mental and manual labour. The

115

democratic-participatory principle referred to the relationship among the staff, between the staff and their pupils, as well as between the school and the parents. Finally, the emphasis on the importance of environment to education was meant to play down the importance of hereditary factors that were then considered paramount in teaching methods. It was not so much a rejection of hereditary factors, as an argument that they are socially produced.

Many Marxists, and indeed non-Marxists, would easily support three of these features of socialist education – universal, participatory and environmentalist. Few contemporary Marxists, however, have taken up the challenge of polytechnical education with its radical implications for the organisation of both schooling and work. There is certainly no mention of polytechnical education in the policies advocated by the British Communist Party. The main demands found in its election manifestos are for comprehensive schooling, nursery schools for all, expansion of higher education, reduction in the size of classes, more and better-paid teachers and the abolition of private schools.[62] Many Marxists would also reject the notion of secular education if it meant that schools should actively promote atheism. They would find the idea of secular education more acceptable if it meant that the school curriculum should not be overburdened with religious teaching.

Marx and Engels were convinced that many of the illnesses and the high morbidity and morality rates among working-class people were due not simply to industrialisation but to capitalist industrialisation. The relentless pursuit of maximum private profit was the root cause. As a result they were confident that in a socialist society illness would decline. It is a view accepted by Marxist writers in the health field today who see socialist medical care as being universal, preventive and participatory. Thus all British Marxist writers are in support of the National Health Service, even though they find it wanting in several respects. The emphasis on prevention is associated with a demand for less technological medicine while the emphasis on participation is linked with a demand for de-professionalisation. Contemporary Marxist writers on health issues, such as Doyal, Carpenter and Navarro, adopt similar positions. After stressing that a socialist form of medical care must go beyond simply asking for more provision along the lines of the National Health Service, Doyal, for example, concludes that

a socialist health service would not only have to provide equal access to medical care but would also have to address itself seriously to such problems as how to demystify medical knowledge and how to break down barriers of authority and status both among health workers themselves and also between workers and consumers.[63]

These demands for participation, de-professionalisation and prevention have been voiced by many non-Marxist authors of whom Illich is perhaps the best known.[64] One of the major differences, however, between the Marxist and non-Marxist is that the latter believe that many of these reforms are possible within the capitalist system while the former insist that only in a socialist society are these possible.

Engels had more to say on housing than Marx but even then it did not add up to much. As with illness, so with bad housing: the root cause lay in the capitalist system and its characteristic form of industrialisation which involved massive rural migrations to towns. In a mature, socialist society 'the modern big cities will be abolished' to be replaced with 'as uniform a distribution as possible of the population over the whole country'.[65] During the very early stages of socialism, however, 'the housing shortage can be remedied immediately by expropriating a part of the luxury dwellings belonging to the propertied classes'.[66] Though neither he nor Marx was prepared to speculate in detail on the actual distribution of housing, it follows from their general writings that in a communist society housing will be communal, it will be provided according to need and it will be democratically administered. Many contemporary Marxists, however, have accepted the argument that owner-occupied housing is so prevalent nowadays among working-class people, that it will be impossible to abolish in a socialist or communist society.[67]

Neither Marx nor Engels said anything about socialist social security apart from stressing that during the transitional stage of socialism adequate provisions should be made 'for people unable to work, etc., in short for what today comes under so-called poor relief'.[68] Under communism, distribution of income would be according to need which would obviate the necessity of a social security system. It was Lenin who made the clearest statement on what a socialist social security system would be like. He set out the following four principles in a speech in 1912:

(i) It should provide assistance in all cases of incapacity including old age, accidents, illness, death of the bread-winner, as well as maternity and birth benefits.

(ii) It should cover *all* wage earners and their families.
(iii) The benefits should equal *full* earnings and *all* costs should be borne by employers and the state.
(iv) There should be uniform insurance organisations (rather than organisations by risk) of a territorial type and under the full management of the insured workers.[69]

Lenin clearly went beyond the existing social security provisions of his time but he did not depart drastically from their underlying assumptions, particularly by his insistence that benefits should be paid only to wage earners, thus excluding the mass of self-employed farmers.

There has been little discussion of a socialist social security system by contemporary Marxist authors and what little there has been does not depart much from Lenin's formulation. Thus, Kincaid insists that a socialist social security system should be universal and financed out of general taxation. Both the insurance principle and means-testing should be abolished because the first excludes many people from receiving benefits while the latter 'is a recipe for the creation of second-class citizens'.[70] Benefits of adequate standard should be paid to all who fall into certain need-producing situations – unemployment, sickness, old age, etc.

In brief, then, Marxists have argued that socialist social services should be focussed ideally on the meeting of need. Second, social services should be universal in coverage not only in their intent but in practice as well. Third, social services should be participatory while the power of the professions should be curtailed as far as possible. Fourth, Marxists see prevention as a vital principle of social services. They urge a departure from the ambulance wagon notion of social services as institutions which sweep up and sort out the problems produced by an economic and social system which neglects human needs. It is for this reason that they feel that truly preventive services cannot be established in a capitalist system.

Thus, certain principles of socialist social policy can be distilled from the Marxist critique of welfare in capitalist society but much work needs to be done to translate them into the basis of a programme. Deacon's work is a start in this area. He acknowledges that there is a need to go beyond general principles to apply them 'to each area of social policy in turn to make concrete our image of the future of social welfare'.[71] Without such development, Marxism will remain a mere form of intellectual activity which is counterproductive to the cause of socialism, for the refusal to tackle practical issues only provides support to the public belief that socialism is nothing but a Utopian dream.

6

The future of the welfare state

In this concluding chapter three rather different tasks are attempted. The first section compares and contrasts the positions of the four groups of thinkers that were considered in detail in earlier chapters. Section II sets out our own perspective on the issues covered in each of the earlier chapters – our view of society and the state, the role of government, our values and our attitude towards the welfare state. The third section reviews some of the lessons learned from the impact of social policy on societies for the future development of the welfare state and outlines a strategy based on the perspective set out in Section II.

Section I The perspectives compared

A close examination of the debates around the values held by the four groups of thinkers reveals one central point: their agreements and disagreements centre fundamentally around their attitudes towards the two related values of freedom and equality. Individualism, pragmatism, humanitarianism, fraternity and other values are important but they are secondary in the sense that they are used to support, to refute, to enlarge or to qualify the values of equality and freedom as perceived by each of the four groups of thinkers.

Freedom is the primary value for the anti-collectivists. They see freedom in negative terms – as the absence of direct coercion of one individual by another or of individuals by governments.

Individuals can be starving but free as well as affluent but unfree. The reluctant collectivists also stress freedom as a central value but it is a different freedom from that stressed by the anti-collectivists. True freedom, as Beveridge pointed out, means freedom from enslavement by want, squalor and other social evils. The anti-collectivists have nothing to say about the coercive power of circumstances or particular patterns of economic and social relationships. The reluctant collectivists, however, do show an awareness of such coercion and of the need for government action to extend freedom.

The Fabians, too, stress freedom as a central socialist value. For them this belief demands a concern to reduce inequality because at certain levels, inequality is a major threat to freedom. This in turn means a belief in government action as a means to creating and increasing freedom – an idea which the anti-collectivists could never accept. As Tawney frequently argued, the increase in the freedom of ordinary men and women in the twentieth century was because of the extended sphere of government activity.

The Marxist notion of freedom is the broadest but the vaguest of all and focusses on the removal of obstacles to human emancipation and self-realisation. If true individual freedom is to be a reality, it must be accompanied not only by a high degree of economic equality but by such an arrangement of economic, political and social relations that individuals can pursue their interests freely within the ideological framework of an altruistic society. It goes beyond the Fabian notion of freedom but, at times, it assumes metaphysical proportions.

These various positions on freedom imply corresponding positions on the value of equality. The anti-collectivists are committed to economic inequality primarily because they believe that any attempts by governments to alter existing patterns of distribution must mean restrictions on individual freedom – their cardinal value. Inequality is therefore necessary to preserve individual freedom but more than that – it is also a necessary precondition for economic growth. Unless people are rewarded as unequally as the private market allows, they will not maximise their efforts to work and to earn, to invest and to save for themselves and their families. The reluctant collectivists, too, believe in the desirability and inevitability of inequality and the preservation of the capitalist system but they want to see current levels slightly reduced for social and humanitarian reasons. In their view, excessive inequalities exacerbate social and political divisions in the country and offend human dignity. They do not

121

see government action to curb excessive inequalities as inimical to individual freedom so long as it is designed to improve the conditions of the lowest paid rather than to promote equality in society in general.

Unlike the anti-collectivists and the reluctant collectivists, Fabians and Marxists see equality as a central value of about equal weight to freedom. Substantial equality of condition makes individual freedom more real, promotes the fulfilment of individual ability and talent, assists social stability and does not undermine work incentives or economic growth. The difference in approach between the two groups of thinkers is not so much over the levels of equality that are considered desirable for they are both fairly unspecific on this. Rather, they differ on the political methods and the pace that they consider possible to reach their objective. Fabians rely totally on the parliamentary road to equality, however long and difficult it may be.

The other values that the various groups support depend very largely on their particular stance towards equality and freedom. Thus it is to be expected that anti-collectivists support individualism, reluctant collectivists espouse pragmatism and Fabians support fellowship.

Though it is true that values can be vague and flexible concepts, there nevertheless exists a large degree of consistency in the various values supported or opposed by the four groups of thinkers. Their value-sets are coherent to a fairly high degree especially when one takes into account the different meaning attached to the same value by the various groups. Values are important for both individuals and for governments. Clearly, no one behaves always according to his or her values but equally, too, no one ignores totally his or her values in everyday life. Governments, too, have to combine the desirable with the possible in their policies and it is no surprise that government rhetoric often differs from government practice. Values are simply one of the many factors that guide practice and it is just as foolhardy to use them as the sole pointer to practice as to ignore them altogether.

Clearly, the values of the four groups of thinkers are related to such important issues in social policy as the models of society espoused, their attitudes to the market system and their views of the state. A discussion of these issues will bring out the essential differences between the four groups towards the welfare state.

The extreme position on society and the state is that of the Marxists who see capitalist society as characterised by inevitable class conflict, conflict which grows out of its basic pattern of economic relations. The Fabians emphasise the reality of class conflict but they do not see it as always and inevitably primary. They emphasise in addition the reality of group conflict which can cut across or override class conflict. The reluctant collectivists have a fundamentally consensus model of society which sees class and group conflict as being erased by economic and social development. The anti-collectivists have virtually nothing to say about class conflict. Their concern is about individual and group conflict but they see the free market system as the great healer of divisions and reconciler of interests rather than as their source.

As pointed out in the first chapter, these divisions of opinion on the nature of society have obvious implications for understanding such issues in social policy as the development of the welfare state, who gains or loses from its operations and its future course. But they also have implications for the understanding of such other important issues in society as racism or sexism. Marxists, for example, will consider sex discrimination as the inevitable result of the class stratification in capitalist societies, while others may see it more in terms of patriarchy, i.e. male domination resulting from a multiplicity of factors over the centuries. These are important issues which space does not allow us to discuss here apart from noting that they need to be given more attention in social policy debates than they have hitherto received.

Attitudes to the free market system differ sharply. For the anti-collectivists, the free market system is the foundation of the self-generating and spontaneous order in social affairs which they regard with such veneration. More specifically, they see the free market system as a vital bulwark of political freedom, as the most efficient system of economic relations yet devised and as the great engine of economic growth. Its success depends only on being left alone by governments once a basic legal and monetary framework has been provided.

The reluctant collectivists accept the effectiveness and validity of the basic capitalist mechanisms but they are sharply critical of unregulated capitalism. In their judgment, capitalism is not, as the anti-collectivists assert, self-regulating. In fact, it will only work well if subject to state regulation. Without such benevolent oversight it is wasteful and inefficient. It fails to use the productive capacity of the economy to the full and it grossly misallocates resources. Of itself, it will not operate so as to abolish injustice and poverty. Furthermore, rather than being a vital foundation for a self-generating and spontaneous political order, it will create conditions directly threatening to political stability if left to operate without government oversight.

The Fabian critique of the free market system is both more complex and sharper. Most Fabians have regarded the private ownership of major enterprises as well as the inheritance of large amounts of capital as unethical. Such a condition perpetuates gross inequalities in society, does not provide adequate opportunities for the fulfilment of ability by all citizens and frequently fails to employ to the full the productive capacity of the economy. It also generates an acquisitive ideology geared to the satisfaction of the desires and demands of individuals to the detriment of communal goals. It is therefore no surprise that advanced welfare capitalist societies combine extreme private affluence with gross public squalor. Nevertheless, Fabians have rarely argued that advanced industrial societies of whatever political system can operate without a substantial money market where individuals can buy the goods and the services that they want.

The Marxist approach to the free market system is sharper than that of the Fabians. They condemn the free market system out of hand as dependent on oppression and exploitation, as underpinning and perpetuating privilege in society and as geared to meeting private demand, however frivolous and ephemeral, at the expense of public needs. They are in favour of wholesale nationalisation programmes, abolition of wealth inheritance and, many of them at least, in favour of confining the operations of the money market to the bare minimum, at least during the communist stage. Free public provision covers a wider range of goods and services than envisaged under any of the strands of Fabianism.

The attitude of the various groups of thinkers towards the state is important because it shows their belief in the possibility of change in the political and economic system. To the anti-collectivists, the state is almost synonymous with the central government which in recent times has been dominated by the power of the electorates. They have been worried by the competitive bidding for votes by governments in parliamentary welfare democracies and by the way in which this makes the governments prisoners of interest groups. It is this feature of the electoral process that has led to excessive government intervention in public affairs. At the other extreme, Marxists define the state in the broadest terms and they see it as substantially, if not totally, constrained by the distribution of economic power in capitalist society and the needs of the capitalist economy. Political and economic moves towards socialism are therefore considered almost impossible through the established parliamentary process. Fabians occupy the middle ground. The state is not simply the creature of dominant economic interests, though their power is acknowledged. It can, therefore, act against their wishes but with great difficulty. Socialist change through the parliamentary process may not be easy but it is possible.

These fundamental differences on the nature of society, the private market and the state inevitably colour the attitudes of the four groups of thinkers towards the welfare state. They range from open hostility to apprehensive acceptance to obvious enthusiasm.

The anti-collectivists are fundamentally hostile to a developed welfare state. Government provision of a basic social minimum is regarded as necessary and relatively unproblematic but provision beyond that is considered both unnecessary and undesirable. Universal and generous government services and benefits have undesirable economic, political and social consequences. Generous government provision has several undesirable economic effects: it diverts human and capital resources from directly productive purposes; it undermines work incentives; and it encourages inefficiency in the administration and consumption of services. Politically, it undermines individual freedom; it ultimately weakens public respect for governments and the political process; and it can thus lead to the emergence of dictatorial regimes. Socially, the more the state gets sucked into the provision of services, the more damage it does to the traditional sources of welfare – the family, the local community and the voluntary agencies. These sources will gradually atrophy – as will people's ability and willingness to provide for their own needs. Anti-collectivists have concentrated their attention on the long-term effects of government provision and they have neglected the short-term blessings and benefits. Even on the consideration of long-term effects, they have ignored totally the Marxist argument that the welfare state has been a major support and benefit to capitalism.

Because they do not share the anti-collectivist anxieties about government action, the reluctant collectivists take quite a different view of the welfare state. They believe governments must act to make good the deficiencies of the free market system and to tackle avoidable ills, though not to bring about major economic and social changes. They therefore consider the welfare state as necessary and beneficial not only to individual people but to the political system as a whole. They are confident that state action can be restricted to combating poverty and that there is no inevitable extension to an attack on inequality, as the anti-

125

collectivists fear. Equally, they are quite happy with a mixed economy of welfare – public, market, voluntary and family. They do not believe that public provision is necessarily destructive of other types of welfare provision. Because of their basic confidence in the market system, they are certain that the state's role will only need to be limited – to make good defects of the free enterprise system.

Fabians are convinced that more will be required of the welfare state than is suggested by reluctant collectivists if life under capitalism is to be tolerable. They have a broader view of the role of public services – to facilitate economic growth, to ease the process of economic and social change, to contribute to social integration, and to reduce inequalities. This broader view is the product of their lesser faith in the ability of the capitalist system to operate efficiently and humanely without government regulation. Above all, however, Fabians see the welfare state not merely as a mechanism for softening the rough edges of an abrasive capitalist system but also as a step – uncertain and tentative certainly – towards a socialist society. Social services are seen as representing a break with pure market doctrines of distribution and as offering evidence to the general public that there is an alternative and effective system of distribution to that of the private market. In recent years, they have been forced by electoral events and by social science evidence to acknowledge that their faith in social services as socialist institutions had been exaggerated. Similarly, their belief that the welfare state as it has operated over the years was a staging post on the road to socialism has been severely tested by recent events in many advanced industrial societies.

Marxists reject the view that the welfare state is a mechanism for changing capitalism. Rather they see the welfare state as a source of support and strength for the capitalist system. It does this by providing services and benefits which make private capital more profitable and which also make the system politically more acceptable – the twin processes of accumulation and legitimation. They accept that in some ways the welfare state does lead to some amelioration of the problems faced by ordinary people but the overall effect is one of economic and political support to the system. Only indirectly do public services provide a threat to political systems – the mounting cost of public services and the consequent problematic faced by governments to raise the required revenues.

To sum up: anti-collectivists see the welfare state as a misnomer. For them, the main source and origin of welfare is the free market system. Anything which threatens that is a source of diswelfare. Reluctant collectivists believe in the necessity and possibility of minor ameliorative state action to ease the pains and injustices of market relations and leave unaffected – or even stronger – the capitalist system in which they believe. Fabians value the welfare state both for what it can and does achieve within a capitalist framework and for gradually providing stepping stones on the road to a socialist order. Marxists are fairly dismissive of this view of the welfare state. They see it as merely providing a short-term but ultimately impermanent solution to the essential contradictions of the capitalist system.

Having compared and contrasted the views of the four groups briefly, we now move to explain in greater detail our own position on these issues and to provide some critical comment on the position of the others.

Section II A critical overview

Apart from the Marxists, the other three groups refer to values as self-contained entities without any real discussion about their origin, how they change or how they relate to the socio-economic system. Marxists prefer the broader notion of ideology which incorporates values, attitudes and beliefs. Though it is not possible to go into these issues in any detail here, a few words of definition and explanation are necessary. Values are implicit or explicit conceptions of what individuals consider to be either ideal ends or desirable means of achieving these ends. The number of such values is limited and, generally speaking, the values held by any one individual – the value set – are congruent with one another to a large extent, though never totally. Contradictions among values are common and, at times, individuals inevitably have to make choices and compromises among their values. In brief, values are generalised cultural ideals which affect people's behaviour in diverse situations and towards different objects. Though people do not always behave according to their value-sets, they are also at times prepared to die for them.

In any society there are certain values which receive general acceptance and support. The value-sets of individuals are variations of this societal value system in the sense that they are neither a mere replica nor completely different from it. Social science debates on the nature of the value system of societies tend to be divided into those which see it as a unitary entity and those which see it as fragmented into various sectional value systems. There has to be a compromise between these two views because if there was a unitary value system in society, one would expect very little social conflict. Everyone in society would be motivated by the same values and conflict would be almost non-existent. On the other hand, if each group in society had its own distinct value system, there would be little agreement in society on anything and conflict would be the rule of the day. All societies have a dominant value system which reflects and supports the existing social order. This dominant value system is perpetuated directly and indirectly, implicitly and explicitly by the various formal and informal institutions of society. Since it reflects the existing social order, the dominant value system inevitably benefits the powerful groups in society most for it endorses existing inequalities. All societies, however, have several sectional value systems reflecting the way of life of major subgroups in society. These sectional value systems incorporate elements of the dominant value system as well as peculiaristic subcultural elements that may be at odds with the dominant value system. These differences, however, are around issues which do not affect the stratification system of society. Thus one does not find subcultural value systems which challenge openly the unequal distribution of economic rewards in advanced industrial societies. Such challenges come from individuals with radical views and not from subcultural value systems.

As mentioned earlier in this chapter, what ultimately divides our four groups of thinkers in their social values is their differing views about freedom and equality. The anti-collectivist and reluctant collectivist view on these two central values represents the dominant value system of society. In other words, inequality is generally accepted in society: it is practised in most aspects of life – at work, at home, at school and elsewhere; and it is eulogised by most social institutions in society – the family, the school, the mass media, the courts, and so on.

The success of the dominant value system has been, first, to convince or simply encourage people to accept the view that inequality is necessary, if not natural, in industrial societies where economic growth is all important. Unless people are paid grossly unequally, they will not strive or work as hard and everyone will thus suffer. Yet there is no evidence to show that those who receive wages that are ten times as high as those of others have either striven or worked harder in their lives. Nor is there any evidence that wage levels are always the sole or dominant attraction to jobs. Nurses' salaries are very low and yet there has never been a shortage of candidates for nurse training. This is not to deny that extra income can motivate people to work harder. Rather it is to suggest that this claim has been exaggerated and that it does not explain existing inequalities – these are based mostly on family background and on professional certification. Above all, too, existing ideologies of work incentives are social constructions and they can be changed.

Second, anti-collectivists have argued that government attempts to reduce inequalities will not only be detrimental to economic growth but they will also destroy individual freedom. Historical evidence in all advanced welfare capitalist societies contradicts this view. It is surely incorrect to argue that individual freedom today is less real than it was at the beginning of the century when government intervention in public affairs was limited. It is equally incorrect to maintain that individual freedom is less real in Sweden than in Japan because the former has a far wider range of government services. In brief, inequality may well be generally accepted but the empirical evidence for its necessity is dubious to say the least. Equality and freedom, as well as equality and economic growth, are not antithetical.

The Fabian and Marxist view that a greater degree of equality enhances individual freedom is supported by both logic and evidence. Where inequality dominates economic relations, it will dominate social and political relations too, and the less well off will be the creatures and victims of the powerful. True freedom depends on a reduction of existing inequalities. It is only through legislation and government action that the freedom of the weaker can be protected against the depredations of the stronger. To enhance the freedom of the majority, the freedom of some members of society will have to be reduced. The final judgment about the desirability of such government action must be about the degree and sum of freedom in society not simply about individual losses or gains. Judged from this perspective, government egalitarian legislation can only enhance the extent of freedom in society. It can help to create a more equal and a freer society where fellowship – concern for one's fellow human beings rather than individualism – influences individual and institutional actions.

In the final section of the chapter, an attempt is made to set out the main conclusion that can be drawn from forty years of welfare statism for a democratic socialist strategy. Before that, however, the structure of society and the nature of the state in advanced capitalist societies are examined in order to provide a clearer picture of the problems and possibilities of such a strategy.

The structure of advanced industrial societies

All advanced industrial societies today exhibit substantial government activity. A high proportion of their income and wealth today is produced directly by government-owned enterprises. A large share of their income is spent by their governments on a wide range of social and public services. A very sizeable section of their labour force is employed by central and local governments. A complex network of rules and regulations control or influence the activities of the private sector. It is this increased government activity – and the speeches of axe-grinding politicians – that has led some commentators to the conclusion that contemporary advanced industrial societies are benevolent 'welfare' states. Heavy emphasis has been placed on the 'welfare' activities of governments while the economic relations used to generate and distribute wealth and income have been substantially ignored. The political system of these societies and the claims they make about themselves have been emphasised at the expense of analysis of the fundamentally unchanged nature of their economic systems.

Contemporary advanced industrial societies are essentially capitalist in nature despite the substantial government activity which characterises them. Private enterprise remains the main source of national wealth and the private market is still the main distributor of national wealth. Government activity normally supplements and supports private enterprise and the private market; it rarely supplants them. Capitalism as an economic system has obviously undergone many changes over recent decades in the ways it is funded, organised and administered, but it has retained its four central features – the private ownership of the means of production and distribution; the maximisation of private profit; the inheritance of substantial amounts of wealth thus perpetuating a largely hereditary capitalist class; and the dominance of an individualistic competitive ethic in economic and social relations.

Welfare capitalism differs in many important respects from *laissez-faire* capitalism but it has not ceased being capitalism. It has been modified, not transformed. The capitalist class which owns most of the means of production and distribution is today larger and less homogeneous than it was in the past. There are more fractions within it today – industrial, commercial, banking, insurance – and they are fractions which do not always have immediate common interests. As a result, there are now more conflicts of interest than in the past, not only between the various fractions of capital but also within them. Thus, though the capitalist class is still in control of the means of production and distribution, it must not be seen as always speaking with one voice on the many issues it has to settle with other elements in society or with the state. If this change has led at times to some weakening of its position, the other major change has had the opposite effect. The growth of national and multi-national enterprises has given the capitalist class immense economic and political power.

In brief, the capitalist class is larger, less homogeneous, more international, subject to more government regulation, but quite as powerful today as in the past. It derives its immense power from various inter-related sources: the ownership of the means of production; the ownership or control of most of the mass media; the common family and educational background shared with other powerful élites in society; and a sustaining dominant ideology. It is now generally acknowledged that the ownership of the means of production means that decisions by large national and international companies can be as, or even more, important than government decisions in relation to employment prospects, wage rises, price increases and related economic issues. The legal freedom of the mass media is undoubtedly an important and valuable asset in welfare capitalist societies but this does not change the simple fact that since most of the media are owned privately, they are more likely to support the interests of private capital than to encourage debate about its nature or to engage in fundamental criticism of its operations. Finally, there is the influence of the dominant ideology in society. Every economic system needs a legitimising ideology and capitalism is no exception. Such values as individualism, inequality, competition, private property are essential to a capitalist economic system and these values are generally accepted and almost universally encouraged by societal institutions. It is as natural for a capitalist economic system to be underpinned by a capitalist set of values as it is for a socialist or a feudal system to have a congruent value-set.

Despite the wide range of government activities today, the working class still largely relies on its labour for its livelihood. This is not to belittle either the importance of public services or the substantial rise in the standards of living of working-class people. It is merely to state a simple fact that is sometimes

131

overlooked. Similarly, the rise in the standards of living should not be confused with reductions of wealth or income inequalities. The top 10 per cent of wealth owners still possess most of the country's wealth and any vertical redistribution that has taken place in the last forty years has mainly been either within the nuclear family or from the very rich to the rich. Similar points could be made to counter the notion that there has been any significant redistribution of income over the years.

What made most change to the lives of ordinary people in the generation after 1945 was the possibility of finding secure employment. Until the late 1970s, such possibilities were far greater than in pre-war days which meant not only a new income security but also the possibility of advancement in life. This change has been accompanied by two other changes – numerical increase in the size of the organised working class, and a growth of factional interests within it. Like the capitalist class, it is larger in size but less homogeneous.

The working class draws its power from three related sources: demand for its labour, organisational unity and political consciousness. When demand for labour is strong, trade unions are also strong and they are more likely to be able to extract high wages from employers. Strength through unity has been a common theme in the development of trade unions and it relates both to the unity of workers within the same trade union as well as the unity between different trade unions. Unity is obviously easier to achieve at times of low rather than high unemployment rates yet its value as a source of power for the working class is more crucial at times when demand for labour is weaker, i.e. at times of high unemployment. Government legislation in relation to trade unions can also have an effect on the organisational unity of trade unions and hence on their power.

The political consciousness of the working class refers both to its willingness to defend the legal rights of trade unions as well as to the political aspirations or voting patterns of working-class people. It is quite possible for workers to be determined defenders of trade union rights without necessarily aspiring to socialist objectives. The history of trade unionism in most countries suggests that though working-class support for trade union rights has not waned over the years, there has been a decline in the general support of the working class for socialist solutions to the problems of capitalism. Thus, trade union policies and claims have become less political over the years and more concerned with immediate issues of wages and hours and conditions of work. It seems that so long as capitalism satisfies the economic aspirations of the working class, it is unlikely that socialism will regain the mass appeal it once had.

No discussion of social class formation in advanced industrial societies is complete which does not incorporate the middle class. Definitional problems abound in this area for it is difficult to draw hard and fast boundaries between the middle class on one hand and its neighbours on the other. Perhaps the best way to understand the position of the middle class in the stratification system is to regard its lower sections as having an economic and political affinity with the working class whilst its more affluent strata should be seen as leaning towards the capitalist class either because of their managerial functions or because of their high professional and economic status, or both. This means that a person's position in the class structure has to take into account not only his relation to the means of production but also the rewards derived from employment – earnings, fringe benefits, job security, general working conditions and career prospects. It complicates the old neat division of society into two classes but it does more justice to contemporary reality. Without this, one is forced into the untenable position of claiming that bank managers and bank cleaners both belong to the working class for they each have to sell their labour for their livelihood.

The analysis presented here argues that conflict of economic interests between the classes is inevitable in advanced industrial societies though the extent and the form it takes have changed over the years. Violent confrontations have generally become rarer and industrial conflict is less often openly combined with political conflict. Institutional arrangements for preventing and resolving strikes have been developed by governments in most countries with varying degrees of success.

Though class conflict remains a fact of advanced industrial societies, it is by no means the only form of conflict in these societies. Conflicts between racial groups, religious groups, status groups and the sexes are also commonplace in varying degrees in different countries. Racial conflicts are perhaps the most prominent as well as the most threatening to social stability in many advanced industrial countries. Religious conflicts are on the wane, largely because of the increased secularisation of society. The rise of the feminist movement has also highlighted situations in which the interests of men and women do not coincide and which lead not to open or violent conflict but to concealed or institutional conflict. Finally, the growth of interest groups has created numerous potential conflict situations – between the various housing tenure groups, between the retired and those at work, and so on.

These types of conflict do not necessarily run along class lines. The conflict of interests between owner-occupiers and council tenants, for example, is not a class conflict because a large proportion of working-class people are owner-occupiers. Similarly, racial conflicts are not always class conflicts. Similar comments apply to an even greater extent in the case of sex and religious conflicts. Thus, all these group conflicts cut across class lines, creating a far more complex web of alignments and confrontations in society. The fundamental difference, however, between class conflict and the various types of group conflict is that, while theoretically at least, the abolition or disappearance of group conflicts is not dependent on the abolition of capitalism, class conflict will only disappear when capitalism itself is transcended.

Clearly, this type of analysis of the structure of contemporary welfare capitalist societies differs fundamentally from that of the anti-collectivists who do not recognise the existence of classes or class conflict, who tend to see trade unions as the most powerful pressure groups and who see conflict as centring around the competition between individuals in society. It is also different from Crosland's post-capitalist view of advanced industrial societies which sees the managers and not the owners of private enterprise as the most powerful group in society, which maintains that private profit maximisation has been replaced by social goals as the *raison d'être* of private enterprise and which sees government regulation of industry as having undermined the power of the capitalist class. Such a view was appealing in the late 1950s and 1960s when economic growth and full employment were common to all advanced industrial countries. Today it has lost all credibility with the spectacle of massive labour redundancies made in order to maximise private profit and with the passing of legislation in many countries that undermines the power of the trade unions.

The traditional Marxist view that sees advanced industrial societies as comprising two monolithic classes and which subsumes all types of conflict under class conflict is also incompatible with the reality of contemporary society. It does not take enough into account the obvious divisions within both capital and labour. Nor does it recognise the often independent existence or importance of group conflicts which are common-place today.

The nature of the state

The analysis of the power structure in society adopted here precludes two of the commonly held views of the nature of the state in advanced industrial societies. It rules out that pluralist conception which sees the state as an independent authority arbitrating impartially between the various contending interest groups and enforcing its decisions without too much difficulty. It rules out, too, the early Marxist view which sees the state as nothing more than a committee that blindly serves the interests of the capitalist class. The pluralist view ignores the very substantial power of private capital while the Marxist view makes it all-powerful at all times and in all situations. The analysis of the power structure in society presented here leads to the rather untidy but realistic notion of the relative autonomy of the state. In other words, the state operates within the structural constraints set by private capital but it always possesses a certain amount of freedom to act independently depending on the nature of the issue, the political ideology of the government, public opinion, and the balance of class forces.

Several of the Marxist writers on the state assume that all issues dealt with by the state are of direct or indirect relevance to the stability and continuation of the capitalist system. A closer analysis of government policies, however, raises serious doubts about this. There is a group of government policies concerning mostly, but not exclusively, moral issues which have nothing to do with the survival of the capitalist system. Examples of this are policies on adoption, abortion, family planning, divorce, capital punishment, drug addiction, and so on. Several other policy areas, too, appear to be equally unrelated to capitalism's survival – policies in relation to parks, sport, cemeteries, sewage, and so on. It is difficult to see how either the form that such services take or the extent of provision has implications for capitalism as a system. At the other extreme, there is a group of policies concerned with clear economic issues which are most relevant to the survival of capitalism – nationalisation of private industry, taxes on wealth, price and wage policies, investment, industrial training, and so on. Such government policies are so obviously relevant to capitalist interests that no elaboration is necessary. Finally, there is a host of other policies with varying degrees of relevance to capitalism. Examples of these in descending order of relevance are social security benefits, education, roads, penal policies, and so on. In this discussion it is also important to point out that because a certain government policy is threatening to the profitability of one particular industry, it does not follow that it is also threatening to the capitalist system as such. Thus, government duties on tobacco and other government measures designed to limit smoking are threatening to the tobacco industry but not necessarily equally threatening to the capitalist system itself.

The political ideology of the government is the second consideration that has to be taken into account in considering the autonomy of the state to act against the interests of the capitalist class. Though the state consists of several agencies – central and local government, civil service, judiciary, the police, the army, social work, and so on – the central government is by far the most important, particularly in parliamentary democracies. It can therefore matter a great deal whether the government is of a Conservative or a Socialist or Social Democratic ideology as far as the type of policies that are pursued. This is not to suggest that socialist governments can ride rough shod over capitalist interests but rather that they are more likely to pursue anti-capitalist policies than other governments. Governments of whatever political ideology must promote economic growth and they have, therefore, to take into account in varying degrees the wishes and the demands of the industrial and business élites. As mentioned earlier, decisions by these élites at the national and international level have profound effects on the employment prospects, wage packets, price levels, and so on in society. Theoretically, however, it is rational to argue that socialist governments are more likely to stand up to such pressures than other governments. Whether they will be successful, even partially, to hold off such pressures depends on several national and international factors which are beyond the scope of this discussion.

The nature of public opinion in parliamentary democracies is the third factor that sets limits to the actions of the state. All governments want to be re-elected and they cannot therefore persistently act against public opinion. Thus, Conservative governments cannot blatantly serve the interest of the capitalist class. They have either to mobilise public opinion in their support or to modify their policies accordingly. Socialist governments are even more hemmed in because of the general pro-capitalist bias of the mass media, the top civil servants and other élites. In brief, the political institutions set some limits to the pro-capital policies of Conservative governments but far more to the radical or reformist policies of socialist governments.

The power of the working class must somehow be brought into the debate on the autonomy of the state. As mentioned earlier, this power has several sources and, when effectively mobilised under favourable circumstances, governments have to take notice of the demands of trade unions. Power is a relational not an absolute concept and when, therefore, the power of the working class is at its peak it follows that the power of the capitalist class is less strong. The balance of class forces in society changes depending on the relative power of the two main classes with corresponding implications for the autonomy of the state.

In brief, then, the state in capitalist societies is more likely to serve the interests of the capitalist than the working class, first, because of the dominant power of that class in economic affairs, second, because of the general bias of the political institutions in a parliamentary democracy that favour conservatism rather than socialist change, and third, because of the generally accepted dominant ideology. This view of the state implies that the parliamentary road to socialism is, at best, gradual and slow, and at worst, uneven and uncertain. There are no inexorable economic or political forces driving welfare capitalism towards socialism. It also means, however, that the extra-parliamentary road to socialism is even less viable for it will be resisted by many sections of the community including some of those who objectively may stand to gain from it. This analysis also implies that attempts by right-wing governments to dismantle universal social services in favour of residual means-tested forms of provision are also unlikely to succeed quickly, if at all, for they face opposition from organised labour, from other sections of the public, from some of the mass media and even from individuals within the capitalist class itself. It is this opposition, and not the fear that such policies will undermine profitability or legitimation of capital, that has so far impeded right-wing governments from 'rolling back the frontiers of the state'. Only periods of very exceptional social and economic upheaval can provide opportunities for governments to move swiftly and substantially towards either socialism or uninhibited *laissez-faire* capitalism. Under other circumstances, political change towards either the left or the right is likely to be gradual and incremental even though the rhetoric may well suggest otherwise.

The welfare state

As pointed out earlier in this chapter, the apprehension and hostility of the anti-collectivists toward the welfare state are based on dogma rather than analysis. There is no real evidence that the expansion of public services has undermined either individual freedom or economic growth. Indeed, all the available evidence strongly suggests that these services and benefits have expanded true individual freedom and have encouraged economic growth by improving the quality of labour, facilitating the mobility of labour and encouraging demand for manufactured goods. Nor is the claim that substantial reductions in social service provision will lead to the family and the local community filling the gap convincing. These two institutions already carry out diverse social service functions but there is both a limit to the burden that can be imposed on them, and there are also some responsibilities which they cannot assume. Thus, many families provide financial support to their members at difficult times but it is unrealistic to expect that they should be obliged to do this at all times and under all circumstances. Similarly, many families care for their elderly members voluntarily and often without state aid but it would be the height of folly to believe that they can be forced to do this all the time. The need for social services has been created through economic, social and demographic changes and the satisfaction of that need cannot be left either to the private market or to the family. Withdrawal of state services will mean that suffering in society will increase very substantially.

The Marxist approach to the welfare state has great strengths and weaknesses. Its strength lies in the way it locates the welfare state within the context of a particular economic and social system rather than seeing it in isolation. Its weaknesses, as we see them, are threefold. First, it sees the effects of social policy in simple mono-directional terms. Because it is based on the theoretical model which sees the state as a mere servant of capitalist interests, it either assumes or it provides partial evidence which shows that social policy acts in one way only – the economic and political support of the capitalist system. Detailed analysis, however, shows that the effects of social policy can be both supportive and undermining of the economic and political system.

The second weakness of the Marxist approach is that it divides the effects of social policy into two more or less separate and equal effects – economic and political. Those services that are said to assist economic growth and profitability are, in fact, indispensable to political legitimation. Put differently, economic growth provides the strongest legitimating force to capitalism. Without the achievement of economic growth, capitalism runs the risk of losing people's allegiances for it has no other major ethical claim. Even the supporters of capitalism have always accepted that its ethical claim lies not in its pursuit of social justice or egalitarianism but in the constant improvement of general living standards. Vice-versa, too, political stability is helpful to the promotion of economic growth and increased profitability.

Third, the Marxist analysis does not bring out well enough the beneficial effects of social policy on the well-being of individual people in terms of income, education, health, housing and general living standards. That has been considerable. It tends to concentrate, at times almost exclusively, on the broader political implications of social policy and it either neglects or denigrates its benefits to individual people and families. Only at times of right-wing attacks do Marxists discover the value of social services and become their staunchest champions.

The Fabian approach towards the welfare state has much to commend it but it also suffers from several weaknesses. The basic Fabian tenet that public and social services provide real benefits to people and that they are worth defending and developing is unquestionably correct. The major weaknesses of the Fabian approach are its unrealistic assumptions that social services are socialist in nature and that the state can be easily turned into a powerful instrument of socialist reform. All the evidence shows that social services confer as many benefits, and sometimes more, on the higher as on the lower socio-economic groups and they have done little to reduce class or gender inequalities in societies. Fabian analysis has also often forgotten the basic fact that the state in welfare capitalism remains a capitalist state and any really reformist government will be constrained by that never-to-be-forgotten fact.

Moreover, the Fabian approach to social problems has relied far too much on centralised, top down, professionally expert services. As a result, it has helped to create services which often serve the interests of the providers as much as those of the users and, on occasions, even more. It is only recently that Fabians have become aware of the need to provide universal services in ways in which they are responsive to the views and demands of their users, particularly at the local level. The customer may not always be right but he is not always wrong either.

How do we view the impact of the welfare state? The major success of the welfare state has been the achievement of certain minimum standards of provision in various aspects of life. It is true that there are still minorities whose incomes are below the official poverty line, who are homeless or whose housing is inadequate, whose health and education services are substandard or who cannot obtain assistance from workers in the personal social services, but this should not be allowed to obscure the fact that for most people in need, social services have proved helpful.

The achievement of minimum standards for most people, however, should not be confused with reductions of class inequalities. As mentioned earlier, the slight redistribution of income and wealth that has taken place in the last forty years has been mainly from the very rich to the rich. Socio-economic differences in adult and infant mortality rates have not narrowed over the years despite the general fall in death rates. Entry to university is as much influenced by family background today as it was in the 1920s, despite the very substantial rise in the number of university students. Social class inequalities in the field of housing remain very wide despite, again, the general improvement in housing standards. Occupational benefits, directly and indirectly encouraged by the state, are still biased heavily in favour of middle- and upper-class groups. In every sphere of social policy that one looks at the picture is very similar: substantial improvement of standards over the years but equally substantial persistence of social class inequalities.

While the impact of social policy on poverty, broadly defined, and inequality is fairly clear, the same cannot be said about its impact on economic development. Separating rhetoric from reality is far more difficult because the evidence is fairly inadequate. Our own evaluation of the empirical evidence led us to the conclusion that social policy has made a net contribution to economic growth, though not as significant as some of the human capital protagonists have sometimes claimed. The contribution of education and training policies, of regional and labour mobility policies to economic growth far outweigh any minor disincentive effects of some of the other aspects of social policy.

A similar conclusion emerges from the equally inadequate evidence on the impact of social policy on political stability: the net effect is support for the existing socio-economic system. Public services do create stresses on the political system because of the problems involved in raising the necessary revenues but, on the other hand, they contribute to political stability in four possible ways: by easing potentially disruptive problems; by adopting individualistic explanations of social problems; by fostering certain values and forms of behaviour; and by helping to replace class conflict with less threatening group conflicts.

Section III The future of the welfare state

The above assessment of the impact of public policy leads to several related conclusions for the future development of the welfare state from a democratic socialist perspective.

The failure of the welfare state to achieve minimum standards for all in the areas covered by social policy will continue in the future however much the services are expanded unless firm legal backing is given to the notion of social rights. This already exists in health and education but it is lacking in social security, housing and various aspects of the personal social services. The argument is that in the same way that an individual has a legal right enforceable in courts of law to health and education services, he should have a legal right to the other services because of his status as a citizen of the country irrespective of such other considerations as work or contribution record, behaviour record or ability to pay. It means, for example, that social security benefits should be financed out of general government revenues in the same way as other public services, and they should be paid to those satisfying certain objective criteria – unemployment, illness, retirement, and so on – without reference to considerations such as work record, behaviour at work or away from work, length of period in need. Similar comments also apply to housing and the personal social services.

This is surely the first and most pressing reform for any democratic socialist government. The present levels of poverty and deprivation in affluent societies are unacceptably high. They are the most painful and damaging of social problems in their effect on people. The reduction of inequalities should be the second area in terms of government priority, though this cannot be achieved through the social services alone. In all welfare capitalist societies, reformist governments since the last war have subscribed to the view that people's incomes from work should, in normal circumstances, be left to the interplay of market forces while the ensuing income inequalities should somehow be reduced through the operation of the tax system and the social services. All the available evidence from many countries now shows that this strategy – if it can be so described – has failed. Direct government intervention in the income distribution process is therefore essential for the reduction of income inequalities – a step which is also a necessary prerequisite to the reduction of inequalities in other aspects of life.

The range of government policies required for the reduction of income inequalities has long been debated among socialists and general agreement exists on most essentials though not on details. Abolition of wealth inheritance is the first step and it has long featured in socialist writings and political pronouncements by Labour or Socialist Parties. There are, however, understandable differences of opinion concerning both the levels of permissible wealth inheritance as well as the appropriate pace and timing of such reforms. Interestingly, abolition of wealth inheritance is also in line with the liberal view of equality of opportunity since it renders the race among competing individuals more equal. Such a reform is not necessarily at odds with a concern for work incentives either since the available evidence shows that about two-thirds of the very rich inherited their wealth. A more equal start in life may well engender more competitiveness among individuals and so provide a greater spur to economic growth.

Securing a less unequal distribution of income, however, will necessitate more government measures than abolition of the inheritance of wealth. Income from work will need to be so distributed that it is sufficient for people's socially agreed needs first, before extra income is distributed according to special need, special merit or special contribution to the common good. In practical policy terms, this means the establishment of both a minimum and a maximum wage and a continuing incomes policy together with adequate child benefits. The exact differentials have to be such as not to undermine work incentives, bearing in mind the present state of the dominant value system. As mentioned earlier, however, too much should not be made of this. The significance of income inequalities for work incentives is much less clear than many supporters of inequality would have us believe. It is the duty of egalitarians continually to question and expose the arguments which are used to bolster existing inequalities of income. The forces that make for value changes in society are complex but one of them is the taking of initiatives in the battle of ideas that is constantly being waged both openly and covertly between radicals and the supporters and beneficiaries of the *status quo*.

A major reduction of income inequalities has implications for other types of inequality and other areas of social policy – none more so than in the area of housing. Government-provided housing will still be necessary for such groups as single people, the temporary, mobile worker, the very elderly, students, those who for a range of reasons, prefer to rent rather than buy, but the majority of the population should be encouraged to buy their own houses. There is no reason why home ownership should be antithetical to the idea of socialism. In fact, the opposite is the case for it provides people with more freedom and greater equality in their lives. The essential thing is that people should be able to afford to buy their house and that the standard of housing should be good enough for all. Inequalities of housing will inevitably remain but they will be nothing like those prevailing today.

Closely related to income inequalities are those in the areas of health and education which have proved so resistant to change over the years. The experience of several countries shows that inequalities in these areas of life can only be reduced by a range of government programmes that go beyond the particular service. What is needed is a health policy not just a health service; an education policy and not merely an education service. Other aspects of life – working and living conditions, income levels and diet patterns, leisure and playing facilities – are highly relevant though outside the present remit of the health or education services.

Evidence from many welfare capitalist societies shows that, at least from the early 1970s onwards, important sections of the public have been critical of the organisational structures of social services – their private and undemocratic decision-making processes, their unresponsiveness to consumer convenience and to public complaints and their over-reliance on professional experts. This has led to demands for greater public participation in the management and organisation of social services – a demand which is very much in accord with the spirit and practice of democratic socialism. Management, through the normal processes of local government, does not guarantee appropriate democratic control. Participation means involvement of actual and potential users and other citizens in the development, organisation and actual running of services. The corollary of this, if it is to become a reality, is a decentralisation and localisation of services. To be a reality participation must be local – at the level of the health centre, the local school, the housing estate, the social services area office, the old people's home.

The case for democratisation and participation combines arguments of principle and practice. The argument of principle is obvious – services for people in a democratic society should involve citizens directly in their running. The argument of practice is that services will be more effective if geared directly to the needs expressed by actual or potential users rather than being based on decisions made by professionals and bureaucrats. There is also the important argument that if popular support is to be maintained for high levels of welfare spending, the citizenry must

143

be kept keenly aware of the extent of social need, the costs of adequate provision for such needs, and of what is being obtained by the expenditure of public funds. If a welfare state is to be transformed into a welfare society, active involvement of citizens is vital. A strategy of decentralisation for democratic participation is essential.

Experiments in participation in social services have shown that the idea is not as simple as many had supposed and that it can bring costs in terms of time and possibly efficiency. Finding the right approach and adapting existing systems and structures is not easy. For example, if users of services are to participate in their organisation and management, this raises very sharply the question of staff participation, which in turn raises questions about traditional patterns of authority in bureaucratic organisations.

We do not ignore these difficulties or the fact that participation means very different things in different situations. All we wish to argue is the necessity to move towards more participative systems on grounds of principle – that is, how things ought to be – and on grounds of practice – that is, the only way to secure flexible, responsive and effective services which sustain public support. Securing participation means major and radical changes in the ethos and structure of services – and it will be opposed (as are all reforms) by those whose convenience and interests are threatened by its introduction and implications.

It has taken the rise of the feminist movement and the election of a right-wing government in Britain to highlight the importance of the so-called informal sector of welfare, particularly in the area of social care. What has emerged is a new emphasis on a pattern of activity which is far from new. The family, the wider kin network, neighbours, friends and voluntary agencies have always been the main providers of care for the elderly and the physically and mentally handicapped.

Feminists have stressed that care by the family and informal sector in fact means care by women and they have emphasised how heavy the burden can be. Right-wing governments have seized on the informal sector as justifying and legitimating cuts in public services and as contributing to the redomestication of women.

A democratic socialist policy must accept the fact that the contribution of the informal sector is vital to the quality of life of many dependent people, that they prefer family care, and that families basically want to provide such care. Such a policy must, however, also take account of what that policy may mean to women and the quality of their lives. For the New Right, the mixed economy of welfare is a euphemism for cuts in public provision. For the socialist, the term describes a new pattern of partnership between statutory and voluntary, formal and informal, family and state welfare. It describes a new orientation in public welfare provision, an orientation which takes account of other vital sources of welfare and which seeks to support and work with them.

A genuine partnership between statutory, non-statutory and family forms of social care is the most effective method of providing adequate services. The core of the partnership, however, must be government commitment to provide the necessary funds and services for otherwise the primary burden will continue to fall on women as unpaid labour. This surely is the fundamental difference in the conception of the mixed economy of welfare from a socialist and a right-wing perspective. There is nothing in socialist ideology that is antithetical either to the family or to the use of volunteers or to community participation in the provision of welfare, provided those offering their services receive support, recognition and, if necessary, payment from the state. A democratic socialist strategy of social care based on these principles is necessary, for there is no doubt that care for special needs groups such as the elderly and handicapped cannot be provided satisfactorily by full-time state employees alone.

The final lesson to have emerged from the operations of the welfare state during the last forty years is that economic and social policy must be looked at together. Economic growth will not, of itself, reduce economic and social inequalities. Reducing inequalities without growth may be possible but it will be extremely difficult. Any economic strategy, therefore, has social implications and, equally, any social strategy depends on assumptions about how the economy functions, and how it will and should function. Thus economic policies during the last forty years, and particularly since the late 1970s, have been more significant in their implications for equality and inequality than social policies. The most striking inequality in society today is between the employed and the unemployed which is the product of particular economic policies. Undoubtedly, too, economic policy has always dominated social policy considerations, with the result that social services have expanded, contracted or stagnated to suit particular economic objectives. It is high time that the relationship between the two types of policy objectives was placed on a more equal footing. Nowhere is this more evident than in the need to develop a policy for work. In the full employment years between 1945 and the early 1970s, governments could, and did, ignore employment policy. It seemed unnecessary when the problem was shortage of labour rather than shortage of work. In the mid-1980s, however, when work has become a scarce commodity, this major aspect of life can no longer be ignored. A policy is needed to create, organise and, if necessary, share work. There will always be some people who can live happy, creative and useful lives without working. That should be welcomed – gratefully – by society when work is short. Most people, however, need to work to have a framework for their lives, a sense of worth and satisfaction, the social contacts which work brings. The absence of work is something which is profoundly damaging to most people and so to society.

If that is accepted, then the provision of work becomes a major responsibility of government. Work sharing may be less 'efficient' in economic terms than a system which allows substantial numbers of the workforce to work long hours of overtime while three or four million people are unemployed. Such an equation cannot be regarded as acceptable. It reflects a narrow and mistaken notion of efficiency. It cannot be regarded as economically or socially efficient in any meaningful way to run the economy in a way which is so wasteful and damaging to so many people.

We accept that such policies for work may have costs. So do current policies, but we need a different and bolder form of social accounting and an approach to the problem which does not clearly disadvantage particular groups. A society such as Britain in the mid-1980s, with more than three million people out of work and a mass of socially worthwhile jobs needing to be done, is obviously a society which has lost its way and has retreated into the obscurantism of economic scholasticism in an attempt to prolong an economic system that is manifestly irrational and detrimental to the welfare of most people.

The analysis of the distribution of power in society and of the nature of the state presented in the second section of this chapter suggested that under normal circumstances radical changes through government policies towards the right, and even more so towards the left, are most unlikely to come about easily or in short periods of time. The failure of the Thatcher government in Britain to move the welfare state towards *laissez-faire* capitalism and of the Mitterand government in France to move towards socialism quickly are evidence of this. It follows that egalitarian governments have no option but to proceed gradually and incrementally. What is more important, however, is that reforms should be treated both as important in themselves and as parts of a wider plan – as stepping-stones on the road to democratic socialism.

Clearly, some of the policies outlined above will be more easily accepted and will face less opposition than others. Thus there is no logical reason why public participation, government commitment and support of the voluntary and family sectors of social care, and even legal backing of social rights, could not be implemented within the economic framework of advanced welfare capitalist societies. Such policies do not pose direct and frontal attacks on the four essentials of capitalism mentioned earlier in this chapter. Reductions of class, gender or race inequalities on the scale suggested above, and the creation of a work policy, however, are direct threats to capitalism and they cannot be implemented within the existing economic framework of advanced capitalist societies. Nor can these policies be achieved under corporatist forms of government which attempt to bring together capital and labour without altering the parameters of capitalism. These policies can only be achieved gradually by democratic socialist governments and they will depend on the assent, albeit reluctant, of capitalist enterprises to the supremacy of social goals or on a planned extension of different forms of social ownership.

The post-war period has witnessed the growth of welfare services in all advanced industrial societies and has, at the same time, exposed the fallacy of the early view that socialism is somehow 'historically inevitable'. No welfare capitalist society today appears to be any closer to democratic socialism than it was in the late 1940s. Yet welfare capitalism cannot be the end of all social evolution, for change is always taking place in society, even though its pace is slow and its direction uncertain. What is certain, however, is that the present social, economic and political problems faced by welfare capitalist societies cannot be managed away by technical or administrative reforms. Nor can they be solved by *laissez-faire* capitalism as the experience of some countries under right-wing governments today shows. Democratic socialist policies are the necessary, if not the sufficient, precondition for the amelioration or solution of many of these problems.

Notes

Chapter 1 Society, the state, social problems and social policy

1 P.S. Cohen, *Modern Social Theory*, Heinemann, 1968, Chs 3-6.
2 R. Dahrendorf, *Class and Class Conflict in Industrial Society*, Routledge & Kegan Paul, 1959, p. 161.
3 T. Parsons, *Sociological Theory and Modern Society*, Free Press, 1969, p. 6.
4 T. Parsons, *Towards a General Theory of Action*, Harvard University Press, 1951, p. 227.
5 D. Lockwood, 'Some Remarks on "The Social System" ', *British Journal of Sociology*, Vol. VIII, No. 2, 1956.
6 A.W. Gouldner, *The Coming Crisis of Western Sociology*, Heinemann, 1971, p. 353.
7 P.L. Van den Berghe, 'Dialectic and Functionalism: Towards a Theoretical Synthesis', *American Sociological Review*, Vol. 28, No. 5, October 1963.
8 K. Davis and W. Moore, 'Some Principles of Stratification', *American Sociological Review*, Vol. 10, No. 2, April 1945.
9 A. Inkeless, *What is Sociology? An Introduction to the Discipline and Profession*, Prentice-Hall, 1964.
10 R. Dubin, 'Approaches to the Study of Social Conflict: A Colloquium', *Conflict Resolution*, Vol. 1, No. 2, June 1957.
11 W.G. Runciman, *Social Science and Political Theory*, Cambridge University Press, 1965, p. 138.
12 M. Weber, *Economy and Society*, New York, 1968, Vol. 2, p. 938.
13 J. Lambert, C. Paris and B. Blackaby, *Housing Policy and the State*, Macmillan, 1978, p. 6.
14 A. Giddens, *Capitalism and Modern Social Theory*, Cambridge

University Press, 1972, p. 156.
15 T. Parsons, 'The Distribution of Power in American Society', *World Politics*, Vol. X, No. 1, October 1957.
16 J.K. Galbraith, *American Capitalism*, Penguin, 1963, p. 125.
17 R.A. Dahl, *Who Governs?*, Yale University Press, 1961, p. 216.
18 P. Bachrach and M. Baratz, *Power and Poverty*, Oxford University Press, 1970.
19 C. Wright Mills, *The Power Elite*, Oxford University Press, 1956.
20 P. Hall, H. Land, R. Parker and A. Webb, *Change, Choice and Conflict in Social Policy*, Heinemann, 1975, pp. 150-2.
21 L. Althusser, *Lenin and Philosophy and Other Essays*, New Left Books, 1971.
22 R. Miliband, *Marxism and Politics*, Oxford University Press, 1977.
23 N. Birnbaum, *The Crisis of Industrial Society*, Oxford University Press, 1969, p. 5.
24 R.A. Nisbet and R.K. Merton, *Contemporary Social Problems*, Harcourt Brace & World, 1966, p. 804.
25 *Ibid.*, pp. 802-3.
26 C. Wright Mills, 'The Professional Ideology of Social Pathologists', *American Journal of Sociology*, Vol. 49, No. 2, 1943.
27 W. Ryan, *Blaming the Victim*, Orbach & Chambers, 1971, p. 27.
28 *Ibid.*, p. 7.
29 J. Horton, 'Order and Conflict Theories of Social Problems as Competing Ideologies', *American Journal of Sociology*, Vol. 71, No. 6, May 1966.
30 J.R. Rule, 'The Problem with Social Problems', *Politics and Society*, Vol. 2, No. 1, 1971.
31 Nisbet and Merton, *op. cit.*, p. 785.
32 G.M. Sykes, *Social Problems in America*, Scot, Foresman, 1971, pp. 9-10.
33 A. Liazos, 'The Poverty of the Sociology of Deviance: Nuts, Sluts and Perverts', *Social Problems*, Vol. 20, No. 1, Summer 1972.
34 I. Taylor, P. Walton and J. Young, *The New Criminology*, Routledge & Kegan Paul, 1973, p. 214.
35 C. Kerr *et al.*, *Industrialism and Industrial Man*, Harvard University Press, 1960.
36 D. Bell, *The End of Ideology*, Free Press, 1960, pp. 402-3.
37 T. Parsons, 'Communism and the West: the Sociology of Conflict', in A. and E. Etzioni (eds), *Social Change*, Basic Books, 1964, p. 397.
38 J. Goldthorpe, 'The Development of Social Policy in England 1800-1914', *Transactions of the Fifth World Congress of Sociology*, Vol. 4, No. 4, 1962, pp. 50-1.
39 W. Moore, 'Functionalism' in T. Bottomore and R. Nisbet (eds), *A History of Sociological Analysis*, Heinemann, 1979.
40 Hall *et al.*, *op. cit.*, p. 150.
41 J. Rex, *Key Problems of Sociological Theory*, Routledge & Kegan Paul, 1961, p. 129.

42 J. Rex, *Social Conflict*, Longman, 1981, p. 47.
43 I. Gough, *The Political Economy of the Welfare State*, Macmillan, 1979.
44 J. O'Connor, *The Fiscal Crisis of the State*, St Martin's Press, 1973.
45 R. Miliband, 'Politics and Poverty', in D. Wedderburn (ed.), *Poverty, Inequality and Class Structure*, Cambridge University Press, 1974, p. 194.
46 R. Quinney, *Class, State and Crime*, Longman, 1977, p. 58.

Chapter 2 The anti-collectivists

1 M. Friedman, *Capitalism and Freedom*, Chicago, 1962, p. 12.
2 G. Dietze, 'Hayek on the Rule of Law', in F. Machup (ed.), *Essays on Hayek*, Routledge & Kegan Paul, 1977, p. 111.
3 F.A. Hayek, *Law, Legislation and Liberty, Vol. I, Rules and Order*, Routledge & Kegan Paul, 1973, p. 61.
4 *Ibid.*, p. 16.
5 F.A. Hayek, *The Constitution of Liberty*, Routledge & Kegan Paul, 1960, reprinted 1976, pp. 20-1.
6 *Ibid.*, p. 137.
7 *Ibid.*, p. 29.
8 Friedman, *op. cit.*, p. 14.
9 F.A. Hayek, *Law, Legislation and Liberty, Vol. 3, The Political Order of a Free People*, Routledge & Kegan Paul, 1979, p. 151.
10 M. and R. Friedman, *Free to Choose*, Penguin, 1980, pp. 181-2.
11 F.A. Hayek, *Individualism and Economic Order*, Routledge & Kegan Paul 1949, p. 22.
12 Quoted in I. Gilmour, *Inside Right*, Quartet, 1978, p. 118.
13 Hayek, *Individualism and Economic Order*, p. 6.
14 *Ibid.*
15 *Ibid.*, p. 13.
16 M. Thatcher, *Let Our Children Grow Tall*, Centre for Policy Studies, 1977, p. 96.
17 F.A. Hayek, *Studies in Philosophy, Politics and Economics*, Routledge & Kegan Paul, 1967, p. 245.
18 *Ibid.*, p. 83.
19 Thatcher, *op. cit.*, p. 81.
20 *Ibid.*, p. 86.
21 A. Gamble, *Britain in Decline*, Macmillan, 1981, p. 150.
22 Friedman, *op. cit.*, p. 195.
23 Hayek, *The Constitution of Liberty*, p. 85.
24 *Ibid.*, p. 87.
25 K. Joseph, *Stranded on the Middle Ground*, Centre for Policy Studies, 1976, p. 62.
26 Hayek, *The Constitution of Liberty*, p. 42.
27 Joseph, *op. cit*, p. 79.
28 Friedman and Friedman, *op. cit.*, p. 176 and p. 178.

29 Hayek, *Law, Legislation and Liberty, Vol. 3*, p. 170.
30 *Ibid.*, p. 150.
31 K. Joseph and J. Sumption, *Equality*, John Murray, 1979, p. 28.
32 Friedman and Friedman, *op. cit.*, p. 177.
33 *Ibid.*, p. 178.
34 Hayek, *The Constitution of Liberty*, p. 83.
35 Friedman and Friedman, *op. cit.*, p. 164.
36 Joseph and Sumption, *op. cit.*, p. 30.
37 F.A. Hayek, *Law, Legislation and Liberty, Vol. 2, The Mirage of Social Justice*, Routledge & Kegan Paul, 1976, p. xi.
38 *Ibid.*, p. 64.
39 Hayek, *Studies in Philosophy, Politics and Economics*, p. 171.
40 *Ibid.*, pp. 66-7.
41 *Ibid.*, p. 136.
42 *Ibid.*, p. 130.
43 Friedman and Friedman, *op. cit.*, pp. 166-9.
44 Hayek, *Studies in Philosophy, Politics and Economics*, pp. 162-6.
45 *Ibid.*, p. 162.
46 F.A. Hayek, *The Road to Serfdom*, Routledge & Sons, 1944, p. 27.
47 *Ibid.*, pp. 151-2.
48 N. Bosanquet, *After the New Right*, Heinemann, 1983, p. 17.
49 Friedman, *op. cit.*, p. 15.
50 Friedman and Friedman, *op. cit.*, p. 21.
51 Joseph, *op. cit.*, p. 57 and p. 62.
52 Bosanquet, *op. cit*, p. 31.
53 Hayek, *The Road to Serfdom*, p. 27.
54 Quoted in W.H. Greenleaf, 'Modern British Conservatism', in R. Benewick, R.N. Berki and B. Parekh, *Knowledge and Belief in Politics*, Allen & Unwin, 1973, p. 204.
55 Friedman, *op. cit.*, p. 15.
56 Friedman and Friedman, *op. cit.*, p. 179.
57 Hayek, *Law, Legislation and Liberty, Vol. 2*, p. 107.
58 Friedman and Friedman, *op. cit.*, pp. 179-80.
59 *Ibid.*, pp. 180-1.
60 Hayek, *Law, Legislation and Liberty, Vol. 2*, p. 139.
61 *Ibid.*, p. 112.
62 A. Seldon, *Wither the Welfare State*, Institute of Economic Affairs, 1981, p. 17.
63 Hayek, *Law, Legislation and Liberty, Vol. 3*, p. 56.
64 *Ibid.*, p. 61.
65 Bosanquet, *op. cit.*, p. 4.
66 Thatcher, *op. cit.*, p. 74.
67 *Ibid.*, p. 73.
68 Hayek, *Law, Legislation and Liberty, Vol. 3*, p. 32.
69 Friedman and Friedman, *op. cit.*, p. 182.
70 Joseph, *op. cit.*, p. 61.
71 Friedman and Friedman, *op. cit.*, pp. 343-7.

72 Hayek, *The Constitution of Liberty*, pp. 107-8.
73 *Ibid.*, p. 110.
74 *Ibid.*, p. 109.
75 S. Brittan, 'The Economic Contradictions of Democracy', *British Journal of Political Science*, Vol. 5, No. 1, 1975, p. 141.
76 *Ibid.*, p. 130.
77 Hayek, *Law, Legislation and Liberty, Vol. 1*, p. 6.
78 Hayek, *Law, Legislation and Liberty, Vol. 3*, p. 129.
79 *Ibid.*, p. 130.
80 A. Gamble, 'Thatcherism and Conservative Politics', in S. Hall and M. Jacques (eds), *The Politics of Thatcherism*, Lawrence & Wishart, 1983, p. 116.
81 E. Powell, *Freedom and Reality*, Elliot Right Way Books, 1969, p. 10.
82 S. Hall, 'The Great Moving Right Show', in Hall and Jacques, *op. cit.*, p. 34.
83 Bosanquet, *op. cit.*, p. 101.
84 Friedman, *op. cit.*, p. 32.
85 Friedman and Friedman, *op. cit.*, p. 24.
86 Friedman, *op. cit.*, p. 3.
87 Hayek, *Law, Legislation and Liberty, Vol. 1*, pp. 132-3.
88 Hayek, *The Constitution of Liberty*, p. 257.
89 D. Heald, *Public Expenditure*, Martin Robertson, 1983, p. 322.
90 Hayek, *Individualism and Economic Order*, p. 110.
91 Hayek, *Road to Serfdom,* p. 29.
92 *The Times*, 2 July 1976.
93 Friedman, *op. cit.*, p. 28.
94 *Ibid.*, p. 30.
95 Hayek, *Law, Legislation and Liberty, Vol. 3*, p. 41.
96 *Ibid.*, p. 42.
97 *Ibid.*, p. 53.
98 Friedman, *op. cit.*, p. 34.
99 Friedman and Friedman, *op. cit.*, p. 53.
100 Thatcher, *op. cit.*, p. 74.
101 N.P. Barry, *Hayek's Social and Economic Philosophy*, Macmillan, 1979, p. 114.
102 F.A. Hayek, *New Studies in Philosophy, Politics and Economics and the History of Ideas*, Routledge & Kegan Paul, 1978, p. 111.
103 Hayek, *The Constitution of Liberty*, p. 285.
104 *Ibid.*, p. 286.
105 Hayek, *Law, Legislation and Liberty, Vol. 3*, p. 55.
106 Hayek, *Law, Legislation and Liberty, Vol. 2*, pp. 142-3.
107 R. Harris and A. Seldon, *Overruled on Welfare*, Institute of Economic Affairs, 1979, p. 204.
108 Seldon, *op. cit.*
109 *Ibid.*, p. 18.
110 Friedman and Friedman, *op. cit.*, p. 249.
111 Hayek, *The Constitution of Liberty*, p. 261.

112 *Guardian*, 26 April 1979.
113 Seldon, *op. cit.*, p. 40.
114 D.S. Lees, *Health Through Choice*, Institute of Economic Affairs, 1961, p. 14.
115 *Ibid.*, p. 30.
116 Friedman, *op. cit.*, p. 186.
117 Friedman and Friedman, *op. cit.*, pp. 146-7.
118 Friedman, *op. cit.*, pp. 147-8.
119 A. Seldon, *Taxation and Welfare*, Institute of Economic Affairs, 1967, p. 68.
120 Friedman and Friedman, *op. cit.*, p. 135.
121 Thatcher, *op. cit.*, p. 83.
122 Seldon, *Wither the Welfare State*, p. 7.
123 Bosanquet, *op. cit.*, p. 162.
124 *Guardian*, 21 January 1981.
125 *Guardian*, 19 January 1981.
126 Friedman and Friedman, *op. cit.*, p. 149.
127 Friedman, *op. cit.*, p. 189.
128 *Ibid.*, p. 155.
129 A. Lejeune (ed.), *Enoch Powell*, Stacey, 1970, p. 32.
130 Hayek, *The Constitution of Liberty*, p. 344.
131 Friedman, *op. cit.*, p. 107.
132 Bosanquet, *op. cit.*, p. 150.
133 Seldon, *Wither the Welfare State*, pp. 12-14.

Chapter 3 The reluctant collectivists

1 D. Heald, *Public Expenditure*, Martin Robertson, 1983, p. 4.
2 Quoted in I. Gilmour, *Britain Can Work*, Martin Robertson, 1983, p. 156.
3 *Ibid.*, p. 69.
4 *Ibid.*, p. 170.
5 W.H. Beveridge, *The Pillars of Security*, Macmillan (New York), 1943, p. 118.
6 J. Harris, *William Beveridge*, Clarendon, 1977, p. 441.
7 J.K. Galbraith, *The New Industrial State*, Deutsch, 1967, 2nd edn, 1972, pp. 363-4.
8 J.K. Galbraith, *Economics and the Public Purpose*, Deutsch, 1974, p. 277.
9 Joan Robinson, 'What has become of the Keynesian Revolution?' in M. Keynes (ed.), *Essays on John Maynard Keynes*, Cambridge University Press, 1975, p. 128.
10 D.E. Moggridge, 'The Influence of Keynes on the Economics of his Time', in M. Keynes (ed.), *op. cit.*, p. 76.
11 W.H. Beveridge, *Full Employment in a Free Society*, Allen & Unwin, 1944, p. 19.
12 *Ibid.*, p. 248.

13 J.K. Galbraith, *The Affluent Society*, Penguin, 2nd edn, 1970, p. 280.
14 R.F. Harrod, *The Life of John Maynard Keynes*, Macmillan, 1951, p. 436.
15 Beveridge, *Full Employment in a Free Society*, p. 21.
16 *Ibid.*, p. 36.
17 W.H. Beveridge, *Why I am a Liberal*, Jenkins, 1945, p. 9.
18 H. Macmillan, *The Middle Way*, Macmillan, 2nd edn, 1966, p. 372.
19 J.M. Keynes, *The General Theory of Employment, Interest and Money* (1936), Macmillan, 1946, p. 380.
20 S.E. Harris, *John Maynard Keynes*, Scribners, 1955, p. 75.
21 W.H. Beveridge, *Voluntary Action*, Allen & Unwin, 1948, p. 320.
22 Beveridge, *Why I am a Liberal*, p. 27.
23 Beveridge, *The Pillars of Security*, p. 42.
24 Harrod, *The Life of John Maynard Keynes*, p. 333.
25 Keynes, *The General Theory*, p. 374.
26 *Ibid.*, p. 373.
27 I. Gilmour, *Inside Right*, Quartet, 1978, p. 179.
28 *Ibid.*, pp. 181-2.
29 *Ibid.*, pp. 114-15.
30 Quoted in D. Reisman, 'Galbraith and Social Welfare', in N. Timms (ed.), *Social Welfare: Why and How*, Routledge & Kegan Paul, 1980, pp. 189-90.
31 D. Owen, *Face the Future*, Cape, 1981, p. 112.
32 W. Rodgers, *The Politics of Change*, Secker & Warburg, 1982, pp. 80-1.
33 *Guardian*, 6 January 1984.
34 Galbraith, *The Affluent Society*, p. 21.
35 *Ibid.*, p. 5.
36 *Ibid.*, p. 98.
37 J.M. Keynes, *The End of Laissez-Faire*, Hogarth (1926), 1927, p. 39.
38 M. Stewart, *Keynes and After*, Penguin, 1967, p. 88.
39 Beveridge, *Full Employment in a Free Society*, p. 29.
40 Galbraith, *The New Industrial State*, p. 225.
41 *Ibid.*, p. 6.
42 *Ibid.*, p. 33.
43 Galbraith, *Economics and the Public Purpose*, p. 179.
44 Quoted in I. Gilmour, *Britain Can Work*, p. 82.
45 Galbraith, *The New Industrial State*, p. 251.
46 *Ibid.*, p. 261.
47 R.F. Harrod, 'Keynes the Economist', in S.E. Harris (ed.), *The New Economics – Keynes' Influence on Theory and Public Policy*, Knopf, 1947, p. 72.
48 Beveridge, *Full Employment in a Free Society*, p. 248.
49 Social Insurance and Allied Services, Cmd. 6404, HMSO, 1942, p. 165.
50 J.M. Keynes, *Essays in Persuasion*, Harcourt, Brace (1931), 1932, p. vii.

51 Galbraith, *The Affluent Society*, p. 212.
52 Galbraith, *Economics and the Public Purpose*, p. x.
53 Galbraith, *The New Industrial State*, pp. 347-8.
54 Social Insurance and Allied Services, p. 166.
55 Galbraith, *The Affluent Society*, p. 105.
56 *Ibid.*, p. 265.
57 Galbraith, *Economics and the Public Purpose*, p. 162.
58 Gilmour, *Britain Can Work*, pp. 224-5.
59 S. Williams, *Politics is for People*, Penguin, 1981, p. 37.
60 D.E. Moggridge, *Keynes*, Macmillan, 1980 (2nd edn),
    p. 46.
61 Beveridge, *Full Employment in a Free Society*, p. 37.
62 *Ibid.*, p. 23.
63 Keynes, *The End of Laissez-Faire*, pp. 52-3.
64 Harris, *John Maynard Keynes*, p. ix.
65 Beveridge, *Full Employment in a Free Society*, p. 206.
66 J.K. Galbraith, *American Capitalism*, Penguin, 1963, p. 185.
67 *Guardian*, 5 April 1974.
68 D. Reisman, *Galbraith and Market Capitalism*, Macmillan, 1980,
    p. 101.
69 P.M. Sweezy, 'Keynes the Economist', in S.E. Harris (ed.), *The
    New Economics – Keynes' Influence on Theory and Public Policy*,
    Knopf, 1947, p. 108.
70 Harris, *William Beveridge*, p. 106.
71 Gilmour, *Inside Right*, p. 118 and p. 151.
72 *Ibid.*, p. 148.
73 Galbraith, *Economics and the Public Purpose*, p. 221.
74 Gilmour, *Britain Can Work*, p. 74.
75 *Ibid.*, p. 168.
76 Reisman, *Galbraith and Market Capitalism*, p. 5.
77 Harris, *William Beveridge*, p. 475.
78 Gilmour, *Britain Can Work*, p. 179.
79 Harris, *William Beveridge*, pp. 433-5.
80 Gilmour, *Britain Can Work*, p. 175.
81 Rodgers, *The Politics of Change*, p. 58.
82 Beveridge, *Why I am a Liberal*, p. 8.
83 Beveridge, *Full Employment in a Free Society*, p. 36.
84 Owen, *Face the Future*, p. 14.
85 A. Smithies, 'Full Employment in a Free Society', *American
    Economic Review*, Vol. 35, 1945, p. 366.
86 Keynes, *The End of Laissez-Faire*, pp. 46-7.
87 Galbraith, *American Capitalism*, p. 94.
88 Keynes, *The General Theory*, p. 380.
89 Beveridge, *Full Employment in a Free Society*, p. 29.
90 *Ibid.*, p. 135.
91 Keynes, *The General Theory*, p. 373.
92 Beveridge, *Full Employment in a Free Society*, p. 186.
93 Stewart, *Keynes and After*, pp. 126-7.

94   Beveridge, *Full Employment in a Free Society*, p. 201.
95   Galbraith, *Economics and the Public Purpose*, p. 213.
96   Gilmour, *Britain Can Work*, pp. 171-9.
97   Owen, *Face the Future*, p. 166.
98   Beveridge, *Full Employment in a Free Society*, p. 186.
99   Beveridge, *Why I am a Liberal*, p. 37.
100 Gilmour, *Inside Right*, p. 151.
101 Quoted in *ibid.*, p. 168.
102 *Ibid.*, p. 152.
103 Harrod, *The Life of John Maynard Keynes*, p. 399.
104 *Ibid.*, p. 535.
105 Beveridge, *The Pillars of Security*, p. 101.
106 Beveridge, *Full Employment in a Free Society*, p. 254.
107 W.S. Churchill, *Liberalism and the Social Problem*, Hodder & Stoughton, 1909, p. 82.
108 Social Insurance and Allied Services, p. 9.
109 Beveridge, *Full Employment in a Free Society*, p. 187.
110 Social Insurance and Allied Services, pp. 95-6.
111 Galbraith, *Economics and the Public Purpose*, pp. 252-3.
112 Social Insurance and Allied Services, pp. 11-12 and p. 108.
113 Beveridge, *The Pillars of Security*, p. 134.
114 Social Insurance and Allied Services, pp. 6-7.
115 *Ibid.*, p. 120.
116 Beveridge, *Full Employment in a Free Society*, p. 256.
117 Social Insurance and Allied Services, p. 12.
118 Beveridge, *Full Employment in a Free Society*, p. 163.
119 Social Insurance and Allied Services, p. 164.
120 Galbraith, *The Affluent Society*, pp. 211-12.
121 Galbraith, *Economics and the Public Purpose*, p. 279.
122 Galbraith, *The Affluent Society*, p. 265.
123 Owen, *Face the Future*, p. 401.
124 *Guardian*, 25 January 1984.
125 Owen, *Face the Future*, p. 388 and p. 393.
126 Gilmour, *Britain Can Work*, p. 152 *et seq.*

Chapter 4 The Fabian socialists

1   B. Crick, 'The Many Faces of Socialism', *New Socialist*, No. 5, May-June 1982.
2   R.N. Berki, *Socialism*, Dent, 1975.
3   C.A.R. Crosland, *The Future of Socialism*, Cape, 1956, p. 113.
4   R.H. Tawney, *The Attack and Other Papers*, Allen & Unwin, 1953, p. 182.
5   M. Meacher, *Socialism With a Human Face*, Allen & Unwin, 1982, p. 239.
6   J.M. Winter and D.M. Joslin, *R.H. Tawney's Commonplace Book*,

Cambridge University Press, 1972, p. 54.
7   Crosland, *The Future of Socialism*, p. 196.
8   *Ibid.*, p. 207.
9   R.M. Titmuss, 'Social Welfare and the Art of Giving', in E. Fromm (ed.), *Socialist Humanism*, Allen Lane, 1967, pp. 358-9.
10 Crosland, *The Future of Socialism*, p. 215.
11 R.H. Tawney, *Equality*, Allen & Unwin, 1931, p. 81.
12 *Ibid.*, p. 113.
13 Crosland, *The Future of Socialism*, p. 295.
14 *Ibid.*, p. 218.
15 *Ibid.*, p. 295.
16 *Ibid.*, p. 296.
17 Meacher, *Socialism With a Human Face*, p. 106.
18 A. Walker, 'Why We Need a Social Strategy', *Marxism Today*, September 1982; P. Townsend, 'Poverty in the '80s', *New Socialist*, No. 1, September-October 1981.
19 Crosland, *The Future of Socialism*, p. 113.
20 R. Jenkins, 'Equality', in R.H.S. Crossman (ed.), *New Fabian Essays*, Turnstile Press, 1952, p. 69.
21 F. Field, *Inequality in Britain*, Fontana, 1981, p. 14.
22 J.M. Winter and D.M. Joslin, *R.H. Tawney's Commonplace Book*, p. 22.
23 C.A.R. Crosland, *Socialism Now*, Cape, 1974, p. 50.
24 Field, *Inequality in Britain*, p. 227.
25 R.H. Tawney, *The Radical Tradition*, Penguin, 1964, p. 169.
26 S.H. Beer, *Modern English Politics*, Faber, 1969, p. 128.
27 Winter and Joslin, *op. cit.*, pp. 12-13.
28 R.H. Tawney, *The Acquisitive Society*, Bell & Sons, 1921, p. 48.
29 R.M. Titmuss, *Commitment to Welfare*, Allen & Unwin, 1968, p. 199.
30 Meacher, *Socialism With a Human Face*, p. 232.
31 E.F.M. Durbin, *The Politics of Democratic Socialism*, The Labour Book Service, 1940, p. 235.
32 Crosland, *The Future of Socialism*, pp. 94-5.
33 Titmuss, *Commitment to Welfare*, p. 114.
34 J. Kincaid, 'Titmuss, The Committed Analyst', *New Society*, 24 February 1983.
35 Tawney, *The Acquisitive Society*, p. 36.
36 Tawney, *Equality*, p. 27.
37 Tawney, *The Acquisitive Society*, p. 40.
38 Tawney, *ibid.*, p. 135.
39 Tawney, *Equality*, pp. 74-7.
40 Tawney, *The Radical Tradition*, p. 173.
41 R. Terrill, *R.H. Tawney and His Times*, Deutsch, 1973, p. 152.
42 C.A.R. Crosland, 'The Transition from Capitalism', in R.H.S. Crossman (ed.), *New Fabian Essays*, Turnstile Press, 1952, p. 42 and p. 46.
43 Crosland, *The Future of Socialism*, p. 116.

44 Crosland, *Socialism Now*, p. 24.
45 Crosland, *The Future of Socialism*, p. 7.
46 Crosland, *Socialism Now*, p. 44.
47 Meacher, *Socialism With a Human Face*, p. 19.
48 Meacher, *ibid.*, p. 29.
49 *Ibid.*, p. 21.
50 *Ibid.*, p. 32.
51 Tawney, *The Acquisitive Society*, pp. 31-2.
52 *Ibid.*, p. 38.
53 R.M. Titmuss, *Essays on the Welfare State*, Allen & Unwin, 1958, p. 31.
54 *Ibid.*, p. 238.
55 Crosland, *The Future of Socialism*, p. 113.
56 Tawney, *The Attack and Other Papers*, p. 97.
57 Tawney, *Equality*, p. 233.
58 Tawney, *The Acquisitive Society*, pp. 97-8.
59 *Ibid.*, p. 121.
60 Crosland, *The Future of Socialism*, p. 324.
61 Meacher, *Socialism With a Human Face*, Chapter 8.
62 Crosland, *The Future of Socialism*, p. 253.
63 E. Luard, *Socialism Without the State*, Macmillan, 1979, pp. 151-2.
64 Crosland, *The Future of Socialism*, p. 303.
65 P. Townsend, *Poverty in the United Kingdom*, Penguin, 1979, p. 926.
66 P. Townsend, 'Poverty in the '80s', *New Socialist*, No. 1, September-October, 1981.
67 Tawney, *Equality*, p. 125.
68 *Ibid.*, p. 133.
69 T.H. Marshall, *Sociology at the Crossroads*, Heinemann, 1963, p. 302.
70 Crosland, *Socialism Now*, p. 194.
71 Titmuss, *Essays on the Welfare State*, p. 39.
72 *Ibid.*, p. 86.
73 Titmuss, *Commitment to Welfare*, p. 191.
74 *Ibid.*, pp. 241-2.
75 R.M. Titmuss, 'Social Welfare and the Art of Giving', p. 359.
76 Tawney, *Equality*, p. 133.
77 Crosland, *The Future of Socialism*, pp. 89-100.
78 T.H. Marshall, *Social Policy*, Hutchinson, 1965, p. 173.
79 P. Wilding, 'Richard Titmuss and Social Welfare', *Social and Economic Administration*, Vol. 10, No. 3, Autumn 1976.
80 R.M. Titmuss, *The Gift Relationship*, Penguin, 1973, pp. 273-4.
81 V. George and P. Wilding, *The Impact of Social Policy*, Routledge & Kegan Paul, 1984, Chapter 1.
82 Titmuss, *Commitment to Welfare*, p. 143.
83 R.M. Titmuss, 'Goals of Today's State', in P. Anderson and R. Blackburn (eds), *Towards Socialism*, Fontana, 1965, p. 357.

84 Titmuss, *Commitment to Welfare*, p. 122.
85 Crosland, *The Future of Socialism*, p. 87.
86 Meacher, 'Socialism With a Human Face', *New Socialist*, No. 4, March-April 1982.
87 Crosland, *The Future of Socialism*, p. 262.
88 R.M. Titmuss, Introduction in R.H. Tawney, *Equality*, Allen & Unwin, 1964 edn, p. 24.
89 Tawney, *Equality*, p. 120.
90 Winter and Joslin, *R.H. Tawney's Commonplace Book*, p. 13.
91 Titmuss, *Commitment to Welfare*, p. 164.
92 Field, *Inequality in Britain*; Townsend, *Poverty in the United Kingdom*.
93 Crosland, *Socialism Now*, pp. 122-3.
94 R.M. Titmuss, *Income Distribution and Social Change*, Allen & Unwin, 1965, p. 188.
95 R.M. Titmuss, 'Goals of Today's Welfare State', p. 362.
96 Crosland, *Socialism Now*, pp. 45-7.
97 Townsend, *Poverty in the United Kingdom*, p. 919.
98 A. Walker, 'Why We Need a Social Strategy', *Marxism Today*, September 1982.
99 Meacher, *Socialism With a Human Face*, Chapter 1.
100 Tawney, *Equality*, p. 219.

Chapter 5 The Marxists

1 F. Hayek, *Individualism and Economic Order*, Routledge & Kegan Paul, 1949, p. 1.
2 K. Marx, 'Preface to a Contribution to the Critique of Political Economy', in K. Marx and F. Engels, *Selected Works Vol. I*, Moscow, n.d., p. 504.
3 R. Miliband, *Marxism and Politics*, Oxford University Press, 1977, p. 10.
4 K. Marx, *The German Ideology*, International Publishers, New York, 1947, p. 22.
5 H. Laski, *A Grammar of Politics*, Allen & Unwin, 1925, p. 149.
6 *Ibid.*, p. 150.
7 J. Strachey, *The Theory and Practice of Socialism*, Gollancz, 1936, p. 198.
8 Miliband, *op. cit.*, p. 190.
9 Laski, *op. cit.*, p. 162.
10 Strachey, *op. cit.*, p. 95.
11 Laski, *op. cit.*, pp. 153 and 154.
12 *Ibid.*, p. 157.
13 *Ibid.*, p. 190.
14 *Ibid.*, p. 194.
15 *Ibid.*, p. 195.

16 *Ibid.*, p. 120.
17 Marx, 'Preface to a Contribution to the Critique of Political Economy', p. 503.
18 F. Engels in his letter to J. Bloch in K. Marx and F. Engels, *Selected Works, Vol. I*, pp. 381-3.
19 H. Laski, *The State in Theory and Practice*, Allen & Unwin, 1934, p. 108.
20 Miliband, *op. cit.*, p. 8.
21 R. Williams, *Culture and Society*, Penguin, 1958, p. 272.
22 P. Taylor-Gooby and J. Dale, *Social Theory and Social Welfare*, Arnold, 1981, p. 185.
23 Laski, *The State in Theory and Practice*, p. 108.
24 K. Marx, *The Eighteenth Brumaire of Louis Bonaparte*, International Publishers, New York, 1969, p. 31.
25 K. Marx, 'Preface to a Contribution to the Critique of Political Economy', p. 278.
26 K. Marx, 'The First International and After', in *Political Writings, Vol. 3*, Pelican edn, London, 1974, p. 324.
27 Laski, *The State in Theory and Practice*, p. 213.
28 Miliband, *op. cit.*, p. 161.
29 D. Coates, 'Reformism', in T. Bottomore (ed.), *A Dictionary of Marxist Thought*, Blackwell, 1983, p. 410.
30 R. Miliband, *The State in Capitalist Society*, Weidenfeld & Nicolson, 1969, p. 12.
31 P. Baran and P. Sweezy, *Monopoly Capital*, Penguin, 1970, p. 40.
32 Miliband, *The State in Capitalist Society*, p. 35.
33 R. Miliband, 'The State', in T. Bottomore (ed.), *op. cit.*, p. 464.
34 F. Engels, 'The Origin of the Family, Private Property and the State', in Marx and Engels, *Selected Works, Vol. 2*, Moscow, 1962, p. 290.
35 Miliband, 'The State', in T. Bottomore (ed.), *op. cit.*, p. 466.
36 R. Miliband, *Marxism and Politics*, Oxford University Press, 1977, p. 69.
37 *Ibid.*, p. 72.
38 R. Mishra, *Society and Social Policy*, Macmillan, 2nd edn 1981, p. 92.
39 L. Althusser, *Lenin and Philosophy and Other Essays*, New Left Books, 1971.
40 A. Barnett, 'Raymond Williams and Marxism', *New Left Review*, No. 99, November-October 1976.
41 J. Strachey, *Contemporary Capitalism*, Gollancz, 1957, p. 180.
42 S. Holland, *The Socialist Challenge*, Quartet Books, 1975, Chapter 2.
43 C.E. Lindblom, *Politics and Markets*, Basic Books, 1977, pp. 122-3.
44 Miliband, *The State in Capitalist Society*, p. 269.
45 F. Engels, *Anti-Duhring*, Moscow, 1954, pp. 305–6.
46 Communist Party of Great Britain, *The British Road to Socialism*,

post 1970 edns.
47 Mary Alice Waters (ed.), *Rosa Luxemburg Speaks*, New York, 1970, p. 391.
48 N. Poulantzas, 'Towards a Democratic Socialism', *New Left Review*, No. 109, May-June 1978.
49 K. Marx, *Capital, Vol. I*, Progress Publishers, 1965, p. 299.
50 Laski, *The State in Theory and Practice*, p. 270.
51 Miliband, *The State in Capitalist Society*, pp. 109-10.
52 E. Mandel, *Marxist Economic Theory*, Merlin Press, 1968, p. 498.
53 Baran and Sweezy, *op. cit.*
54 N. Ginsburg, *Class, Capital and Social Policy*, Macmillan, 1979, p. 2.
55 I. Gough, *The Political Economy of the Welfare State*, Macmillan, 1979, p. 64.
56 *Ibid.*, p. 65.
57 J. O'Connor, *The Fiscal Crisis of the State*, St Martin's Press, 1973, p. 6.
58 Gough, *The Political Economy of the Welfare State*, p. 152.
59 C. Offe, 'Some Contradictions of the Modern Welfare State', *Critical Social Policy*, Vol. 2, No. 2, Autumn 1982.
60 V. George and N. Manning, *Socialism, Social Welfare and the Soviet Union*, Routledge & Kegan Paul, 1980, p. 65.
61 K. Marx, *Capital, Vol. I*, Penguin, 1976, p. 530.
62 Communist Party of Great Britain, *People Before Profits*, 1970, p. 12.
63 L. Doyal, *The Political Economy of Health*, Pluto Press, 1979, p. 294; see also V. Navarro, *Social Security and Medicine in the USSR*, Lexington Books, 1977, p. 118; M. Carpenter, 'Left Wing Orthodoxy and the Politics of Health', *Capital and Class*, Vol. II, 1980.
64 I. Illich, *Medical Nemesis*, Calder & Boyars, 1975.
65 F. Engels, *The Housing Question*, Lawrence, 1942, p. 96.
66 *Ibid.*, p. 77.
67 N. Ginsburg, 'Home Ownership and Socialism in Britain', *Critical Social Policy*, Vol. 3, No. 1, Summer 1983; M. Cowling and S. Smith, 'Home Ownership, Socialism and Realistic Socialist Policy', *Critical Social Policy*, No. 9, Spring 1984.
68 K. Marx and F. Engels, *Selected Works*, Lawrence & Wishart, 1970, p. 318.
69 V.I. Lenin, *Collected Works, Vol. 17*, Foreign Languages Publishing House, 1963, p. 476.
70 J.C. Kincaid, *Poverty and Equality in Britain*, Penguin, 1973, p. 235.
71 B. Deacon, 'Social Administration, Social Policy and Socialism', *Critical Social Policy*, Vol. 1, No. 1, Summer 1981.

Bibliography

Althusser, L., *Lenin and Philosophy and Other Essays*, New Left Books, 1971.

Anderson, P. and Blackburn, R. (eds), *Towards Socialism*, Fontana, 1965.

Bachrach, P. and Baratz, M., *Power and Poverty*, Oxford University Press, 1970.

Baran, P. and Sweezy, P., *Monopoly Capital*, Penguin, 1970.

Barnett, A., 'Raymond Williams and Marxism', *New Left Review*, No. 99, November-October 1976.

Barry, N.P., *Hayek's Social and Economic Philosophy*, Macmillan, 1979.

Beer, S.H., *Modern English Politics*, Faber, 1969.

Bell, D., *The End of Ideology*, Free Press, 1960.

Benewick, R., Berki, R.N. and Parekh, B., *Knowledge and Belief in Politics*, Allen & Unwin, 1973.

Berki, R.N., *Socialism*, Dent, 1975.

Beveridge, W.H., *The Pillars of Security*, Macmillan (New York), 1943.

Beveridge, W.H., *Full Employment in a Free Society*, Allen & Unwin, 1944.

Beveridge, W.H., *Why I am a Liberal*, Jenkins, 1945.

Beveridge, W.H., *Voluntary Action*, Allen & Unwin, 1948.

Birnbaum, N., *The Crisis of Industrial Society*, Oxford University Press, 1969.

Bosanquet, N., *After the New Right*, Heinemann, 1983.

Bottomore, T. and Nisbet, R. (eds), *A History of Sociological Analysis*, Heinemann, 1979.

Bottomore, T. (ed.), *A Dictionary of Marxist Thought*, Blackwell, 1983.

Brittan, S., 'The Economic Contradictions of Democracy', *British Journal of Political Science*, Vol. 5, No. 1, 1975.

Carpenter, M., 'Left Wing Orthodoxy and the Politics of Health', *Capital and Class*, Vol. II, 1980.

Churchill, W.S., *Liberalism and the Social Problem*, Hodder & Stoughton, 1909.

Cohen, P.S., *Modern Social Theory*, Heinemann, 1968.

Communist Party of Great Britain, *People Before Profits*, 1970.

Cowling, M. and Smith, S., 'Home Ownership, Socialism and Realistic Socialist Policy', *Critical Social Policy*, No. 9, Spring 1984.

Crick, B., 'The Many Faces of Socialism', *New Socialist*, No. 5, May-June 1982.

Crosland, C.A.R., *The Future of Socialism*, Cape, 1956.

Crosland, C.A.R., *Socialism Now*, Cape, 1974.

Crossman, R.H.S. (ed.), *New Fabian Essays*, Turnstile Press, 1952.

Dahl, R.A., *Who Governs?*, Yale University Press, 1961.

Dahrendorf, R., *Class and Class Conflict in Industrial Society*, Routledge & Kegan Paul, 1959.

Davis, K. and Moore, W., 'Some Principles of Stratification', *American Sociological Review*, Vol. 10, No. 2, April 1945.

Deacon, B., 'Social Administration, Social Policy and Socialism', *Critical Social Policy*, Vol. 1, No. 1, Summer 1981.

Doyal, L., *The Political Economy of Health*, Pluto Press, 1979.

Dubin, R., 'Approaches to the Study of Social Conflict: A Colloquium', *Conflict Resolution*, Vol. 1, No. 2, June 1957.

Durbin, E.F.M., *The Politics of Democratic Socialism*, The Labour Book Service, 1940.

Engels, F., *The Housing Question*, Lawrence, 1942.

Engels, F., *Anti-Duhring*, Moscow, 1954.

Engels, F., 'The Origin of the Family, Private Property and the State', in Marx and Engels, *Selected Works, Vol. 2*, Moscow, 1962.

Etzioni, A. and Etzioni, E. (eds), *Social Change*, Basic Books, 1964.

Field, F., *Inequality in Britain*, Fontana, 1981.

Friedman, M., *Capitalism and Freedom*, Chicago, 1962.

Friedman, M. and Friedman, R., *Free to Choose*, Penguin, 1980.

Fromm, E. (ed.), *Socialist Humanism*, Allen Lane, 1967.

Galbraith, J.K., *American Capitalism*, Penguin, 1963.

Galbraith, J.K., *The Affluent Society*, Penguin, 2nd edn, 1970.

Galbraith, J.K., *The New Industrial State*, Deutsch, 1967, 2nd edn, 1972.

Galbraith, J.K., *Economics and the Public Purpose*, Deutsch, 1974.

Gamble, A., *Britain in Decline*, Macmillan, 1981.

George, V. and Manning, N., *Socialism, Social Welfare and the Soviet Union*, Routledge & Kegan Paul, 1980.

George, V. and Wilding, P., *The Impact of Social Policy*, Routledge & Kegan Paul, 1984.

Giddens, A., *Capitalism and Modern Social Theory*, Cambridge University Press, 1972.

Gilmour, I., *Inside Right*, Quartet, 1978.

Gilmour, I., *Britain Can Work*, Martin Robertson, 1983.

Ginsburg, N., *Class, Capital and Social Policy*, Macmillan, 1979.

Ginsburg, N., 'Home Ownership and Socialism in Britain', *Critical Social Policy*, Vol. 3, No. 1, Summer 1983.

Goldthorpe, J., 'The Development of Social Policy in England 1800-1914', *Transactions of the Fifth World Congress of Sociology*, Vol. 4, No. 4, 1962.

Gough, I., *The Political Economy of the Welfare State*, Macmillan, 1979.

Gouldner, A.W., *The Coming Crisis of Western Sociology*, Heinemann, 1971.

Hall, P., Land, H., Parker, R. and Webb, A., *Change, Choice and Conflict in Social Policy*, Heinemann, 1975.

Hall, S. and Jacques, M. (eds), *The Politics of Thatcherism*, Lawrence & Wishart, 1983.

Harris, J., *William Beveridge*, Clarendon, 1977.

Harris, R. and Seldon, A., *Overruled on Welfare*, Institute of Economic Affairs, 1979.

Harris, S.E., *John Maynard Keynes*, Scribners, 1955.

Harris, S.E. (ed.), *The New Economics – Keynes' Influence on Theory and Public Policy*, Knopf, 1947.

Harrod, R.F., *The Life of John Maynard Keynes*, Macmillan, 1951.

Hayek, F.A. *The Road to Serfdom*, Routledge & Sons, 1944.

Hayek, F.A., *Individualism and Economic Order*, Routledge & Kegan Paul, 1949.

Hayek, F.A., *The Constitution of Liberty*, Routledge & Kegan Paul, 1960.

Hayek, F.A., *Studies in Philosophy, Politics and Economics*, Routledge & Kegan Paul, 1967.

Hayek, F.A., *Law, Legislation and Liberty, Vol. 1, Rules and Order*, Routledge & Kegan Paul, 1973.

Hayek, F.A., *Law, Legislation and Liberty, Vol. 2, The Mirage of Social Justice*, Routledge & Kegan Paul, 1976.

Hayek, F.A., *New Studies in Philosophy, Politics and Economics and the History of Ideas*, Routledge & Kegan Paul, 1978.

Hayek, F.A., *Law, Legislation and Liberty, Vol. 3, The Political Order of a Free People*, Routledge & Kegan Paul, 1979.

Heald, D., *Public Expenditure*, Martin Robertson, 1983.

Holland, S., *The Socialist Challenge*, Quartet Books, 1975.

Horton, J., 'Order and Conflict Theories of Social Problems as Competing Ideologies', *American Journal of Sociology*, Vol. 71, No. 6, May 1966.

Illich, I., *Medical Nemesis*, Calder & Boyars, 1975.

Inkeless, A., *What is Sociology? An Introduction to the Discipline and Profession*, Prentice-Hall, 1964.

Joseph, K., *Stranded on the Middle Ground*, Centre for Policy Studies, 1976.

Joseph, K. and Sumption, J., *Equality*, John Murray, 1979.

Kerr, C., *et al.*, *Industrialism and Industrial Man*, Harvard University Press, 1960.

Keynes, J.M., *The End of Laissez-Faire*, Hogarth, 1927.

Keynes, J.M., *Essays in Persuasion*, Harcourt Brace, 1932.

Keynes, J.M., *The General Theory of Employment, Interest and Money*, Macmillan, 1946.

Keynes, M. (ed.), *Essays on John Maynard Keynes*, Cambridge University Press, 1975.

Kincaid, J.C., *Poverty and Equality in Britain*, Penguin, 1973.

Kincaid, J., 'Titmuss, The Committed Analyst', *New Society*, 24 February 1983.

Lambert, J., Paris, C. and Blackaby, B., *Housing Policy and the State*, Macmillan, 1978.

Laski, H., *A Grammar of Politics*, Allen & Unwin, 1925.

Laski, H., *The State in Theory and Practice*, Allen & Unwin, 1934.

Lees, D.S., *Health Through Choice*, Institute of Economic Affairs, 1961.

Lejeune, A. (ed.), *Enoch Powell*, Stacey, 1970.

Lenin, V.I., *Collected Works, Vol. 17*, Foreign Languages Publishing House, 1963.

Liazos, A., 'The Poverty of the Sociology of Deviance: Nuts, Sluts and Perverts', *Social Problems*, Vol. 20, No. 1, Summer 1972.

Lindblom, C.E., *Politics and Markets*, Basic Books, 1977.

Lockwood, D., 'Some Remarks on "The Social System" ', *British Journal of Sociology*, Vol. VIII, No. 2, 1956.

Luard, E., *Socialism Without the State*, Macmillan, 1979.

Machup, F. (ed.), *Essays on Hayek*, Routledge & Kegan Paul, 1977.

Macmillan, H., *The Middle Way*, Macmillan, 2nd edn, 1966.

Mandel, E., *Marxist Economic Theory*, Merlin Press, 1968.

Marshall, T.H., *Sociology at the Crossroads*, Heinemann, 1963.

Marshall, T.H., *Social Policy*, Hutchinson, 1965.

Marx, K., *The German Ideology*, International Publishers, New York, 1947.

Marx, K., *Capital, Vol. I*, Progress Publishers, 1965.

Marx, K., *The Eighteenth Brumaire of Louis Bonaparte*, International Publishers, New York, 1969.

Marx, K., 'Preface to a Contribution to the Critique of Political Economy', in Marx and Engels, *Selected Works, Vol. I*, Moscow, n.d.

Marx, K., 'The First International and After', in *Political Writings, Vol. 3*, Pelican edn, London, 1974.

Marx, K., *Capital, Vol. I*, Penguin, 1976.

Marx, K. and Engels, F., *Selected Works*, Lawrence & Wishart, 1970.

Meacher, M., 'Socialism With a Human Face', *New Socialist*, No. 4, March-April, 1982.

Meacher, M., *Socialism With a Human Face*, Allen & Unwin, 1982.

Miliband, R., *The State in Capitalist Society*, Weidenfeld & Nicolson, 1969.

Miliband, R., *Marxism and Politics*, Oxford University Press, 1977.

Mishra, R., *Society and Social Policy*, Macmillan, 2nd edn, 1981.

Moggridge, D.E., *Keynes*, Macmillan, 1980 (2nd edn).

Navarro, V., *Social Security and Medicine in the USSR*, Lexington Books, 1977.

Bibliography

Nisbet, R.A. and Merton, R.K., *Contemporary Social Problems*, Harcourt Brace & World, 1966.

O'Connor, J., *The Fiscal Crisis of the State*, St Martin's Press, 1973.

Offe, C., 'Some Contradictions of the Modern Welfare State', *Critical Social Policy*, Vol. 2, No. 2, Autumn, 1982.

Owen, D., *Face the Future*, Cape, 1981.

Parsons, T., *Towards a General Theory of Action*, Harvard University Press, 1951.

Parsons, T., 'The Distribution of Power in American Society', *World Politics*, Vol. X, No. 1, October 1957.

Parsons, T., *Sociological Theory and Modern Society*, Free Press, 1969.

Poulantzas, N., 'Towards a Democratic Socialism', *New Left Review*, No. 109, May-June 1978.

Powell, E., *Freedom and Reality*, Elliot Right Way Books, 1969.

Quinney, R., *Class, State and Crime*, Longman, 1977.

Reisman, D., *Galbraith and Market Capitalism*, Macmillan, 1980.

Rex, J., *Key Problems of Sociological Theory*, Routledge & Kegan Paul, 1961.

Rex, J., *Social Conflict*, Longman, 1981.

Rodgers, W., *The Politics of Change*, Secker & Warburg, 1982.

Rule, J.R., 'The Problem with Social Problems', *Politics and Society*, Vol. 2, No. 1, 1971.

Runciman, W.G., *Social Science and Political Theory*, Cambridge University Press, 1965.

Ryan, W., *Blaming the Victim*, Orbach & Chambers, 1971.

Seldon, A., *Taxation and Welfare*, Institute of Economic Affairs, 1967.

Seldon, A., *Wither the Welfare State*, Institute of Economic Affairs, 1981.

Smithies, A., 'Full Employment in a Free Society', *American Economic Review*, Vol. 35, 1945.

Social Insurance and Allied Services, Cmd. 6404, HMSO, 1942 (*Beveridge Report*).

Stewart, M., *Keynes and After*, Penguin, 1967.

Strachey, J., *The Theory and Practice of Socialism*, Gollancz, 1936.

Strachey, J., *Contemporary Capitalism*, Gollancz, 1957.

Sykes, G.M., *Social Problems in America*, Scot, Foresman, 1971.

Tawney, R.H., *The Acquisitive Society*, Bell & Sons, 1921.

Tawney, R.H., *Equality*, Allen & Unwin, 1931.

Tawney, R.H., *The Attack and Other Papers*, Allen & Unwin, 1953.

Tawney, R.H., *The Radical Tradition*, Penguin, 1964.

Taylor, I., Walton, P. and Young, J., *The New Criminology*, Routledge & Kegan Paul, 1973.

Taylor-Gooby, P. and Dale, J., *Social Theory and Social Welfare*, Arnold, 1981.

Terrill, R., *R.H. Tawney and His Times*, Deutsch, 1973.

Thatcher, M., *Let Our Children Grow Tall*, Centre for Policy Studies, 1977.

Timms, N. (ed.), *Social Welfare: Why and How*, Routledge & Kegan Paul, 1980.

Titmuss, R.M., *Essays on the Welfare State*, Allen & Unwin, 1958.

Titmuss, R.M., *Income Distribution and Social Change*, Allen & Unwin, 1965.

Titmuss, R.M., *Commitment to Welfare*, Allen & Unwin, 1968.

Titmuss, R.M., *The Gift Relationship*, Penguin, 1973.

Townsend, P., *Poverty in the United Kingdom*, Penguin, 1979.

Townsend, P., 'Poverty in the '80s', *New Socialist*, No. 1, September-October 1981.

Van den Berghe, P.L. 'Dialectic and Functionalism: Towards a Theoretical Synthesis', *American Sociological Review*, Vol. 28, No. 5, October 1963.

Walker, A., 'Why We Need a Social Strategy', *Marxism Today*, September 1982.

Waters, Mary Alice (ed.), *Rosa Luxemburg Speaks*, New York, 1970.

Weber, M., *Economy and Society*, New York, 1968.

Wedderburn, D. (ed.), *Poverty, Inequality and Class Structure,* Cambridge University Press, 1974.

Wilding, P., 'Richard Titmuss and Social Welfare', *Social and Economic Administration*, Vol. 10, No. 3, Autumn 1976.

Williams, R., *Culture and Society*, Penguin, 1958.

Williams, S., *Politics is for People*, Penguin, 1981.

Winter, J.M. and Joslin, D.M., *R.H. Tawney's Commonplace Book*, Cambridge University Press, 1972.

Wright Mills, C., 'The Professional Ideology of Social Pathologists', *American Journal of Sociology*, Vol. 49, No. 2, 1943.

Wright Mills, C., *The Power Elite*, Oxford University Press, 1956.

Subject index

Name index